Dealing with Different Types of Losses Using Hypnotherapy Scripts

Dealing with Different Types of Losses Using Hypnotherapy Scripts is a unique practical resource for hypnotherapists which considers many aspects of loss rather than focusing solely on dying, death and bereavement. It presents new ways of looking at loss and from many different perspectives.

Hypnotherapists will be encouraged to reflect on their own attitudes, values and ways of working on a one-on-one basis and in groups. Loss is inherently important because it can be identified when therapy is already underway and sometimes when it was not the original problem presented to the hypnotherapist. The author is a registered hypnotherapist who has put together a comprehensive range of tried and tested scripts and visualisations for both adults and children (age 5+). The scripts offer a variety of methods to choose from such as: solution-focused, metaphors (Ericksonian), Gestalt therapy, benefits approach and regression. The appendices include an assortment of practical resources and materials, such as: exercises, handouts, questions, forms for the hypnotherapist to use for notetaking during sessions and for developing plans after a hypnotherapy session has taken place.

The book will be of use to students, newly qualified and experienced hypnotherapists and trainers working in hypnotherapy training schools.

Jacki Pritchard, MA, works as a clinical hypnotherapist, independent social worker and trainer in social care. She offers hypnotherapy services to adults and children (age 5+) in two practice locations, schools and colleges.

Dealing with Different Types of Losses Using Hypnotherapy Scripts

Jacki Pritchard

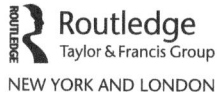
Routledge
Taylor & Francis Group

NEW YORK AND LONDON

Cover image: © Getty Images

First published 2022
by Routledge
605 Third Avenue, New York, NY 10158

and by Routledge
4 Park Square, Milton Park, Abingdon, Oxon OX14 4RN

Routledge is an imprint of the Taylor & Francis Group, an informa business

British Library Cataloguing-in-Publication Data
A catalogue record for this book is available from the British Library

Library of Congress Cataloging-in-Publication Data
Names: Pritchard, Jacki, author.
Title: Dealing with different types of losses using hypnotherapy scripts / Jacki Pritchard.
Description: Abingdon, Oxon ; New York, NY : Routledge, 2022. | Includes bibliographical references and index.
Identifiers: LCCN 2021059355 (print) | LCCN 2021059356 (ebook) | ISBN 9781032245690 (hardback) | ISBN 9781032244129 (paperback) | ISBN 9781032245706 (ebook)
Subjects: LCSH: Grief therapy. | Loss (Psychology) | Hypnotism--Therapeutic use.
Classification: LCC RC455.4.L67 P75 2022 (print) | LCC RC455.4.L67 (ebook) | DDC 616.89/162--dc23/eng/20220404
LC record available at https://lccn.loc.gov/2021059355
LC ebook record available at https://lccn.loc.gov/2021059356

ISBN: 978-1-032-24569-0 (hbk)
ISBN: 978-1-032-24412-9 (pbk)
ISBN: 978-1-032-24570-6 (ebk)

DOI: 10.4324/9781032245706

Typeset in Times New Roman
by Taylor & Francis Books

This book is dedicated to everyone I have worked with and lost over the years – children and adults – you all taught me something for which I am eternally grateful. Also for Georgios and Morgana – who will never be lost.

Contents

Part I

Working with losses

1 Introduction

Hypnotherapy and losses

My background

I suppose in some ways I take the subject of loss for granted because it has always been an intrinsic part of my working life as a social worker and a hypnotherapist. I started my career in social work as a trainee social worker in a children's hospital. I worked on a ward for children who had been diagnosed with leukaemia, other forms of cancer or had brain tumours. Many of my clients died as medical knowledge was not as advanced as it is nowadays. At that time dealing with death was a huge part of my working life. It made me question lots of things – my own beliefs, values and goals. Looking back I know it grounded me and made me the practitioner I am today. Once I qualified as a social worker I worked generically, so I saw both children and adults experience all types of losses. Then I specialised in abuse issues and have done so for the past 40 years; loss for victims is a common experience and so a constant theme in the work I have done in the past and continue to do so – in both my roles as a social worker and hypnotherapist.

The idea for the book

It was a returning hypnotherapy client that made me realise the need for this book; that is, a book which considers different types of losses. People tend to lump together the terms 'loss', 'grief' and 'bereavement'. In my practice as a hypnotherapist, I find that when a client realises that hypnosis really does work if you are motivated to face issues and make changes in your life, s/he often returns for a 'top-up' session if another issue arises for him/her. I had worked with Ms A twice before; hypnotherapy had been effective in helping her deal with people and difficult relationships when she was at University and her lack of confidence. When she came back for the third time (two years on from when we first met) it was just after the first lockdown in England, which happened between March and July 2020. The Covid-19 pandemic presented a difficult time for everyone in a variety of ways. When Ms A contacted me she said she just wanted to talk about

DOI: 10.4324/9781032245706-2

how she was feeling in the first session rather than engage in hypnotherapy, because she felt each member of her family had their own problems and she could not offload how she was feeling on to them. She believed that her problems were less important than those of other family members and she did not want to burden them. Ms A talked for one and a half hours. As she talked it became crystal clear to me how much she had had to endure due to the large number of losses she had experienced – loss of a six-year relationship with her boyfriend; two suicides within the family; and loss of a job opportunity abroad (due to Covid-19). What was so fascinating to me was that Ms A had not connected the fact that she had experienced so many losses in such a short space of time (less than a year).

When I was writing up my notes after the session, it made me reflect on the fact that this can be common for a number of clients, that is, not acknowledging the losses they have experienced or the impact of those losses. It is especially the case for those who do not value themselves and always put others' needs before their own. Somehow the losses are minimised, thought to be of little importance or significance. In fact it is often an indicator of just how resilient people can be. I also think that we still live in a society that finds it difficult to face loss, grief and bereavement head on. Massive steps forward have been made in the past few decades, but many people still think we should show the 'stiff upper lip' and 'just get on' or 'move on'. This is very unhealthy – everyone needs to grieve for any loss they experience. As human beings, we all experience masses of losses – big and small, significant and insignificant; and probably do not think about them a lot of the time. We just assume they are part of life's journey.

I ended up spending ages writing up Ms A's notes from that session. She had got me thinking not only about my hypnotherapy clients I have seen in recent years, but I started reflecting back on my social work clients. I got side-tracked from writing up Ms A's notes and started making a list of all the losses my clients from over the decades had experienced; this included both children and adults. I added to the list over the following few days too as things kept coming back to me. It became an exceedingly long list. I always carry a notebook in my handbag, so I can write down reflective thoughts, ideas, quotes or other random things which may prove useful sometime in the future. In addition to the list of losses clients had experienced, I started writing a separate list of losses which I have personally experienced. For the next few days my mind kept going back to the theme of losses. So this is how I came to realise that it would be useful to put together a book about losses for hypnotherapists.

The Covid-19 pandemic and losses

At that time in 2020, the Covid-19 pandemic had already started to affect people and whilst putting this book together I have become even more conscious of the devastating effects this virus has had around the world. The pandemic has caused a lot of losses in many diverse ways. Obviously, it has caused the death of millions, but in addition people have felt they have lost their freedom. Some people have felt trapped in their households during lockdowns when they have been told to stay home, work from home, shield or self-isolate. Some might argue they have lost their human rights (e.g. life; choice) with being told by politicians what they can and cannot do.

People have been affected physically by the pandemic in all sorts of ways, but mental health has also been affected. We know that the incidence of abuse has increased as people have been stuck living together 24 hours a day, seven days a week. Victims may have experienced physical abuse as well as psychological abuse. Some families have been living in very overcrowded conditions. People have lost their jobs, or had reduced income that has caused worry about being able to provide for their family. It is important to remember that some people are living in poverty or are homeless, which makes them very vulnerable. All these different situations can affect one's mental health and wellbeing. It is very common to hear people talking about:

- Feeling low; lethargic; having no energy or enthusiasm to do anything
- Seeing no end to it all
- Loss of hope; loss of optimism
- Things will never being the same again.

The pandemic will continue to affect the world and there will be an ever increasing need to deal with the losses caused by the pandemic.

Loss, grief and bereavement

Helping clients deal with loss can be a huge part of a hypnotherapist's working life, but very often the subject of loss is not given enough attention in its own right. As already stated above loss, grief and bereavement as subject areas are often lumped together and I understand perfectly well why that happens. However, perhaps it is to the detriment of the different types of losses as people do tend to think about death and dying when the word 'loss' is mentioned. Hypnotherapists like social workers (and other professionals working in the caring professions) are going to work with clients who experience so many different types of loss but I do not think enough attention is given to this in training for hypnotherapists.

Hypnotherapists may work with a client who has deficits in their life, that is, a lack of something (e.g. lack of confidence or self-esteem); the client may say they have never been a confident person and could experience anxiety. A deficit is different to a loss. A client may have been very confident and assertive previously then something happened which caused them to lose these attributes. Of course hypnotherapy can be used to build that confidence and assertiveness again, but work must also be undertaken on dealing with the loss and how it affected and made the client feel and behave. Hypnotherapists will have many skills and techniques in their toolkit, which they can utilise to deal with the effects of any loss a client has experienced. What I wanted to do was to produce a book which would stimulate a hypnotherapist to think more in-depth about the different types of losses and have a resource of scripts to hand which could be utilised in conjunction with the techniques they already use.

Objectives of the book

The main objectives of the book, which is primarily for hypnotherapists (whether a student, newly qualified or experienced) are to:

- Focus on and consider the subject of loss: meaning; all the different types; the effects and consequences of experiencing a loss
- Introduce aspects of loss which a hypnotherapist may never have thought about, considered before or about which they have little/no knowledge
- Be more pro-active in working with losses, that is, not just when a loss arises with a client who is already having hypnotherapy sessions
- Think about what services they might offer in the future: individual/ group work; working in organisations, institutions, specialist facilities
- Become more prepared to work with a variety of losses
- Develop skills in working with losses
- Have a resource of scripts (for both adults and children) which have been tried and tested
- Stimulate ideas (and suggest resources) for Continued Professional Development (CPD).

The journey of grief

A term I use throughout the book is the 'journey of grief'. A person who experiences a loss will deal with it in his/her own way, but may need help in doing this. It is a bespoke journey; nobody can plan in advance the right route to take. The book focuses very much on dealing with emotions along the journey and facilitating travelling towards the final destination i.e. accepting the loss and living life in a new, purposeful way. The book is divided into the following parts:

  (I) Working with losses
 (II) Dealing with emotions
(III) Facing and dealing with death
(IV) Moving forward
 (V) Additional scripts.

In the following chapter more information is given about the content of the parts and there is a guide so that the hypnotherapist can find appropriate scripts easily. I have included scripts for both adults and children (age 5+). Some of the scripts written for adults can be used for young people and children if the hypnotherapist adapts the language so it becomes age appropriate. I have also included scripts, which are specifically for children.

Ways of working with loss: one-to-one or group sessions

I wanted to discuss ways of working right at the beginning of the book because many of the scripts can be used/adapted for group work. I would encourage hypnotherapists to think more about the services they want to offer in the future and I want to promote the idea of 'dealing with losses' groups, so we can move away from thinking about stereotypical bereavement groups. In some circumstances it can be useful to use the term 'grief groups'. Terminology is important and I want loss and losses to be considered in their own right rather than automatically being associated with death.

Working with a loss could arise for the hypnotherapist in a number of ways. A potential client could make contact specifically to ask about help with a loss or bereavement. I think what probably happens more frequently is that the hypnotherapist finds him/herself working with a loss when a client has already started hypnotherapy sessions but had actually presented with a completely different problem. The client may talk about a loss in passing or it might be identified as the root cause of the presenting problem(s). Whatever the situation, the hypnotherapist has to consider the best way of working with a client. For most cases, the hypnotherapy sessions will be conducted on a one-to-one basis (either face-to-face or remotely; the latter more so since the advent of the Covid-19 pandemic) but the hypnotherapist might also consider group work. Some hypnotherapists may decide to run a group and advertise for clients who have experienced some type of loss. In my practice as both a social worker and a hypnotherapist, I have sometimes found that clients I am working with have a specific problem/issue in common and I have then decided to set up a specific group for them. I mention this because it is very relevant for people who have experienced specific losses; some examples being people who have:

- Been a victim of a particular category/form of abuse[1]
- Been a victim of crime (e.g. mugging; burglary; identity theft; bank account hacked)
- Lost their job (e.g. been sacked; made redundant; taken retirement or forced to take early retirement)
- Been caring for someone who is terminally ill.

It is also worthwhile for the hypnotherapist to think about where s/he can provide group work and approach organisations/establishments, for example:

- Schools; colleges and universities
- Children's residential homes
- Young offender units; prisons
- Day care facilities
- Care/nursing homes
- Hospitals
- Hospices
- Local community groups/centres.

If the hypnotherapist decides to run a group for people who have experienced some type of loss then some thought should be given to the following subjects before planning to set up and run such a group[2]:

- Why do I want to run a group?
- Who is the group for?
- What types of losses will be considered/worked on?
- What is the main purpose of the group? (e.g. counselling; therapy; mutual support; other objectives)
- Do I actually have the skills to run a group? Or do I need to undertake some specialised training?
- Will the group be time-limited or an open/ongoing group?
- If the group is time-limited, how many sessions will there be?
- How many people will be in the group? (consider minimum and maximum numbers)
- Where will I run the group?
- What equipment might I need for group work?
- When will the sessions run? (day/night/time)
- Duration of the sessions
- Frequency of the sessions
- Fees/deposits/methods of payment
- Structure of the sessions (e.g. how much time will be allocated for talking in the conscious state; how much time for trance work)
- Content (presentations; information/handouts; how the hypnotherapy will be delivered; methods; techniques; use of scripts).

Whichever way the hypnotherapist decides to work, s/he will find appropriate scripts and visualisations to deal with loss in the chapters which follow. Chapter 2 explains how the book is laid out and includes a guide, so the hypnotherapist can easily and quickly find a script to suit the needs of their client.

Notes

1 There are four categories of child abuse – physical, sexual, neglect and emotional; and ten forms of adult abuse – physical, psychological, financial/material, neglect/act of omission, sexual, discriminatory, domestic violence, modern slavery, organisational and self-neglect.
2 The reader may find it useful to read Chapter 4 'Running groups' in Pritchard, J. (2022) *Hypnotherapy for Pregnancy and Birthing: Scripts for Hypnotherapists.* Abingdon, Oxon: Routledge.

2 How to use the book

Introduction

The book is full of scripts which have a range of objectives and uses to deal with various types of losses. Therefore, it is imperative that a hypnotherapist can find their way around the book easily and not have to spend ages looking for what they need. Obviously the contents and index can be used, but the purpose of this chapter is to briefly explain how the book has been divided up into parts and then to include a guide to the chapters and scripts. I want to state at the outset that scripts have been included for both adults and children (age 5+). Some scripts have been specifically written for children; a number of others can be adapted by simplifying some of the language.

The parts

What follows is a brief summary of what each part in the book covers.

I. Working with losses

The first part of the book explains the purpose of the book and discusses different types of losses, so that the reader is immediately stimulated to think of losses in a broader sense, that is, not just in relation to dying and death. Undertaking a thorough assessment is a crucial part of a hypnotherapist's work. Before any hypnotherapy actually starts, it is necessary to spend time assessing and then to develop a treatment plan. This is discussed in relation to a client but also in relation to a hypnotherapist needing to reflect on his/her own experiences, attitudes and any personal unresolved issues. Two introductory scripts are provided for a first session.

II. Dealing with emotions

The journey of grief is a term which is used throughout the book and in the scripts. The concept of this journey is introduced in this part and the first two chapters include scripts which can be used in a first session to introduce the

DOI: 10.4324/9781032245706-3

client to the journey. The scripts and visualisations presented have the primary aim of dealing with emotions that can result from any type of loss and helping a client to work through their feelings as these emotions arise on the journey of grief. It is emphasised throughout that the journey will be very individual and there is no particular timescale which has to be followed.

III. Facing and dealing with death

Although the book aims to look at different types of losses, it did need to include a section on dying and death. In this part, scripts are included so that a hypnotherapist can work with a terminally ill person (adult or child) and help them to plan for their death. Other scripts are for clients who have been bereaved and need help working through their grief; or for those who struggle to remember a person (e.g. what they looked like; the sound of their voice). Remembrance and commemoration are considered and scripts are included to facilitate this.

IV. Moving forward

The scripts in this part are for use when a lot of the hypnotherapy has taken place and the work is almost complete, that is, the journey of grief is reaching the end (as is the treatment plan). The scripts should be used for acceptance work and moving positively towards the future. Some scripts have been included to deal with any final issues that might still be causing some confusion about the future. However, the main objective is to plan for the future.

V. Additional scripts

This part includes additional scripts which can be used on the journey of grief. Some of the chapters address particular subjects, all of which are related in some way with losses: freedom; assertiveness; human rights; forced marriage.

Using the scripts

As has been mentioned already the scripts can be used/adapted for both adults and children, when working on an individual basis. All the scripts were originally written for face-to-face hypnotherapy sessions but since the Covid-19 pandemic many hypnotherapists have been working remotely. I believe the scripts can be used if a hypnotherapist chooses to work remotely in the future. I also think that some scripts are suitable for use in a group.

The scripts offer a variety of methods to choose from:

- Solution-focussed
- Metaphors (Ericksonian)

- Gestalt therapy
- Benefits approach
- Regression.

Where one or more scripts are presented in a chapter, I have written an introduction at the beginning to explain the purpose and how they should be used. Some introductions are longer than others as some scripts need more explanation. Some chapters include additional scripts, visualisations or appendices with practical resources/materials (e.g. exercises, handouts summary of questions and forms).

Thorough preparation and rehearsal are vitally important before using a script. The hypnotherapist should read, interpret and become familiar with a script before presenting it in his/her own way (maybe having made some adaptations to suit the client). S/he will do this by thinking about the use of:

- Voice
- Tone
- Pitch
- Emphasis
- Pace
- Pauses and silences.

Hence why I have not written within the scripts which words need emphasis or where pauses or silences should occur. The hypnotherapist needs to work with and respond to the client during a session, i.e. work in a person-centred way and go at their pace. Instead I have included *guidance notes* within body of the scripts and at points suggest prompts and/ or questions, which the hypnotherapist can choose to use or not.

Guide to the chapters/scripts

The guide should be used to find an appropriate script/subject area.

---

1. Introduction: Hypnotherapy and losses	*Explains the objectives of the book.*
2. How to use the book	
3. Different types of losses	*Lays the foundations for thinking about the different types of losses which a hypnotherapist may have to work with. Discusses in full the grouping of losses used in the book.*
Appendix 3.1: Summary of different types of losses	

4. Assessment before working with losses	*Discusses the importance of assessment before developing a treatment plan. How assessments can be undertaken.*
Appendix 4.1: Questionnaire for general assessment/loss/bereavement/terminal illness	
Appendix 4.2: Form for exercise – identifying losses	
Appendix 4.3: Form for significant dates	
5. Two scripts for the first session	
Script 1: An introduction to trance	*Gets the client into trance. Relaxation. Creates a peaceful place. Introduces the concept of the journey of grief.*
Script 2: Magic carpet	*Demonstrates the power of the subconscious mind, travelling in the imagination and being in control. Can be used for practising self-hypnosis. For use in future sessions to forward pace or for regression purposes.*
6. Journey of grief	*Discusses/references traditional works and stages of grief. Introduces the concept of the journey of grief. Includes five visualisations which help the client to understand the emotions and pain they may face on their own journey (e.g. difficulty in facing things; bumpy ride; despair, anger; avoidance/denial).*
7. Tour bus	*For use in a first or second session after initially introducing the journey of grief. Demonstrates that there may be things to see, experience, obstacles and detours along the way. The tour guide on the bus is the subconscious mind. Can be returned to in future sessions to work on issues as they arise on the journey of grief (e.g. blockages; uncertainty; lack of direction; things that need to be thrown away/finished with; impatience; frustration; anger).*
8. Lost and found	*To help the client identify exactly what they have lost and what they have found so far on their journey of grief. Useful for reviewing a treatment plan.*
Appendix 8.1: Possible objectives for a client to work towards (in a treatment plan)	
9. Visualisations for emotional pain	*Short general introductory script for visualisations. Seven visualisations to work on emotional pain. To acknowledge and accept that the pain will subside.*

10. It's OK to feel ...

Emphasises the fact that many different emotions/feelings can be experienced on the journey of grief. There is no right or wrong way to feel. Facilitates work on emotions/feelings being experienced.

Appendix 10.1: Emotions and feelings

11. Opening tulips

Relaxation. Openness. To encourage the client to open up about how they are feeling. To encourage discussion about difficult topics or to talk to/confront certain people. Promotes optimism and looking to grow, flourish and thrive.

12. Feeling alone

For anyone who is experiencing loneliness or isolation having been bullied, harassed or is living in new circumstances. Works on developing courage and leaving loneliness behind. A sense of belonging and being part of something is experienced.

13. Fire and anger

To encourage the venting of anger. To deal with the emotion of anger through the use of fire and then to end it.

Script 1: Blazing trail of fire

Script 2: The cremation

14. Learning to cry

To facilitate crying when a client finds it difficult to express emotion or talk about feelings.

Script 1: Dambusters

Script 2: The crying doll

15. Wobbling

Relaxation. Deepening. Letting things happen naturally through learning to wobble. For a client who is struggling to remember specific things about a person who has left, is missing or has died.

16. Icicles

For a client who is emotionally stuck. To get rid of negative feelings and enabling the client to move forward.

17. Ice skating

To demonstrate learning new skills and building confidence during the journey of grief. Suggests the idea there may be some stumbles, slips, trips and falls along the journey. Promotes the idea of recovery, restoration, and balance in life.

18. Dig it up

To help a client talk about anything they have kept to themselves (e.g. thoughts, feelings) or have been avoiding/denying recently or from the past (e.g. people, situations). To bring forward issues buried in the subconscious mind.

19. Trees

Using the image of trees to heal from grief.

Script 1: Fell those feelings

To get rid of feelings.

Script 2: Fallen tree	*To grow new roots and become grounded.*
Script 3: Leaves falling with regrets	*To let go of regrets.*
20. Building and breaking down walls	
Script 1: Building a wall	*To stop recurring or intrusive thoughts.*
Script 2: Breaking down a wall	*For use when a client is blocked or resistant to change; and cannot see any hope for the future.*
21. Leaving the darkness in the cave	*For a client who feels in a dark place; and feels trapped or overwhelmed by his/her thoughts, feelings or current situation. To work on the past if required. To move forward out of the darkness.*
22. Deflation, restoration and improvement	*For a client who is feeling let down or struggling with confidence/learning. To restore former strength; purpose; trust in people and in oneself. To build confidence and self-belief.*
Script 1: For adults – the lilo	
Script 2: For children – swimming ring and arm bands	
23. Egg timer	*A way of making time pass more quickly or more slowly.*
24. Planning for death	*To help a terminally ill client prepare for his/her death. To develop a death plan; what the client wants to happen (what should or should not be said or done) before and after the death. Can be used for a healthy client who wants to plan for their eventual death.*
Appendix 24.1: Questionnaire for developing a death plan	
25. Man in the corner	*Written for a child who is terminally ill. Objective to relax and experience the feeling of being peaceful and not afraid.*
26. Animal heaven	*For a child who has experienced a death of an animal. To embed the idea the animal is now living somewhere else and is not coming back.*
Location 1: Farm	
Location 2: Circus	
Location 3: Zoo	
Location 4: Any other place	
27. Conversations on the clouds	*Relaxation and deepener. Sometimes chosen as a safe place. To talk about and work on regrets. Can be used to rehearse conversations in order to get answers.*

28. The great pyramid

Relaxation and deepener. For a bereaved person to work on remembrance, commemoration and to deal with any unresolved issues.

Additional script 1: Remembering

Additional script 2: Commemorating

Additional script 3: Meeting the deceased person

29. The storage unit

Creating a place to retrieve and store positive memories about a person after a relationship has ended. Can also facilitate regression work.

30. The red admiral butterfly

Metaphorical story about a woman who believes her deceased husband comes back to visit her as a butterfly.

31. Acceptance and aspirations

To commend the client. Review progress. Work on acceptance. Identify hopes and aspirations for the future.

Appendix 31.1: Aspirations – questions, list and plan

32. Preparing for the future

To be used towards the end of a treatment plan in order to plan how the future should be having dealt with the loss.

Script 1: Bumper cars

Reviews progress through the journey of grief and discovers if any other issues need to be bumped out the way before driving into the future.

Script 2: Bungee jumping into the future

Seeing the future and making changes to achieve future hopes and aspirations.

33. The jigsaw puzzle

For working with a client who is feeling unclear, muddled or puzzled about what the future might look like. Fitting pieces together to form a picture of the future.

34. Kaleidoscope

To identify repeating patterns – negative thoughts, feelings, behaviours – habits. To make changes for the future using images in the kaleidoscope. Embeds the idea of change, movement, shifting and enlightenment.

35. Clouds coming together

For use at the end of the journey of grief. To achieve the merging of the past and the present in order to move on to the future.

36. Time capsule

To remember the positive things and times after a relationship has ended badly. To remember the positives, create good memories and to store them in a time capsule which can be returned to in the future.

37. Brightness on the horizon

To work on despair. To give hope and encourage optimism. Looking to the future.

Script 2: For an adult

46. Positivity	*To be used with a client who is presenting as very negative and/or is resistant to making changes.*
Script 1: Signs on the blackboard	*To erase negative thoughts/feelings and multiply positivity.*
Script 2: Good comes out of bad	*To teach that something positive can come out of a negative experience. To unlearn the habit of having a negative attitude to everything.*

3 Different types of losses

There are numerous books written about loss, grief and bereavement and those three words –loss – grief – bereavement – are often put together and considered as one subject area. I explained in the first chapter of this book how working with a particular client had made me reflect on the subject of losses and had inspired me to put this book together. After that session I thought a great deal about the fact that losses can occur regularly in everyday life and an individual human being experiences so many losses through a lifetime. Consequently, some losses are not given any attention at all because they are considered to be a normal part of life. A human being can build resilience – it is a natural response; losses can be seen as part of life's great tapestry. Consequently, some losses and the effects on an individual can be embedded in the subconscious mind and at some point will need to be faced and worked on.

Hypnotherapists will deal with different types of losses in their everyday work with clients. Embedded losses can be identified when a client is in trance; often this can be a total surprise to the client. When they are training, hypnotherapists learn numerous methods of working and techniques; and with practice and experience will probably come to favour a particular way of working. Although finding and using the best method for the client has to be of paramount importance – not what the hypnotherapist prefers to use. Adopting a flexible approach to the work is imperative for hypnotherapy to be effective. As a social worker, I have always favoured adopting the psychodynamic approach to my work, that is, believing that what has happened in the past is vital to understanding the client. In order to move forward the past has to be dealt with. I adopt the same approach in my hypnotherapy practice and favour using regression techniques. Some hypnotherapists do not believe looking back to the past is necessary and will adopt the solution-focussed approach or cognitive behavioural therapy. A properly trained hypnotherapist will have lots of resources (knowledge and skills) in their toolkit and should be able to work with any loss, which is presented to them by a client in a hypnotherapy session. One of the objectives of this book is to stimulate the hypnotherapist to think more in-depth about losses and be prepared for

DOI: 10.4324/9781032245706-4

working with a loss rather than just responding as the need arises in the therapy room.

The purpose of this chapter is to explore the different types of loss that a human being might experience. Below I want to focus on the different types of losses by giving an overview of losses which could be presented to the hypnotherapist (although obviously not every single loss can be highlighted).

Some dictionary definitions of loss

I think with any subject it is always useful to consult the dictionaries and get some definitions in order to reflect on meaning. Here are some definitions of loss and losses:

- the fact that you no longer have something or have less of something
- a disadvantage caused by someone leaving or by something being taken away
- the death of a person

(Cambridge English Dictionary)[1]

- the fact or process of losing something or someone
- the feeling of grief after losing someone or something of value
- a person or thing that is badly missed when lost

(Oxford Compact English Dictionary)[2]

- loss is the fact of no longer having something or having less of it than before

(Collins English Dictionary)[3]

- destruction, ruin
- the act of losing possession
- a person or thing or an amount that is lost
- failure to gain, win, obtain, or utilize

(Merriam-Webster)[4]

- the act or instance of losing
- the condition of being deprived or bereaved of something or someone
- the harm or suffering caused by losing or being lost

(The Free Dictionary)[5]

Broad groupings

I have already stated above that there are just so many losses that could occur in life and it would be impossible to list or discuss them all in this chapter. When I started listing losses after my session with my client, Ms

A, it developed into an exercise that went on for days and I could have continued for much longer but stopped myself. Since then I have developed some broad groupings for the purposes of this book and chapter. Types of losses are divided into:

- People
- Animals/pets
- Relationships
- Objects/possessions
- Health/wellbeing
- Purpose
- Time/stages in life
- The future.

People

The most obvious loss is one of people. People usually think of death in the first instance but through life a person can have many people coming into and going out of their lives – on a personal level or through education/work. One can lose a:

- Relative
- Friend
- Neighbour
- Fellow classmate/student
- Colleague
- Acquaintance
- Person in a position of trust/authority
- Professional/worker/carer/volunteer/befriender.

A change in circumstances can result in a person leaving – maybe through no choice of their own. A person may have to move away physically (e.g. for a job) and although it may be possible to keep in touch remotely with all the technology that now exists (by phone, computer, text, email etc.) but it is just not the same as having the personal face-to-face contact and the familiar routines, meet-ups, activities can be lost. Clients will often state that they did not know how much someone meant to them or how much they relied on them until s/he had left. A loss can become very significant and emotionally painful a long time after the person has left (a year or more later).

There will be situations where a person may choose to leave someone and this ends in separation or a divorce. The hypnotherapist could be working with the person who has been left and consequently s/he is bereft, angry or experiencing a whole gamut of emotions. Alternatively a person who has left a person behind could seek the help of a hypnotherapist because they regret their decision and miss the person they left; or they are experiencing feelings of guilt.

Another aspect of people leaving which hypnotherapists need to consider is missing people – both children and adults. In 2019/2020, there were a total of 325,171 missing person incidents reported in England and Wales; 198,943 related to children and 126,228 adults related to adults.[6] Children sometimes decide to leave home and there could be all sorts of reasons for this. Adults go missing too. The statistics for this year indicate that more males than females went missing; and 319 transgender individuals were recorded as missing persons incidents. Not knowing where someone is can feel unbearable. This could go on for years and sometimes the person never comes back or is never found.

As a social worker, I am very aware of forced marriage situations. People who refuse to have an arranged marriage can be punished because they have brought shame on the family and community. There are cases where such individuals disappear and are never seen again. Such disappearances are rarely reported to the police by family members. A hypnotherapist could work with someone who left home when they were younger (as a child or an adult) and subsequently suffered various traumas – perhaps whilst living on the streets – but later they feel they lost their home and family and need to address this. Missing people may present as clients themselves at any stage of their life. The people who have been left behind could also present for help; either initially when the person has gone missing or later (months/years) when trying to come to terms with what happened.

A person can be lost through the doing of others. Bullying is a very good example of this. In the school/college situation children and young adults can fall in and out of friendships. This can happen when physically attending school but nowadays so much bullying can occur via social media and friendship groups which are formed. It must be acknowledged that adults can also be bullied, for example, in the workplace, social groups/clubs or again via social media. Whilst considering the actions of others, it is important to recognise too that in the extreme a person can be murdered.

When thinking about loss of people, death has to be mentioned. People can die in many different circumstances:

- Suddenly/unexpectedly
- Expected
- Natural causes
- Illness
- Accident
- Suicide
- Murder.

I think it is important to mention that some hypnotherapists, including myself, do work in schools and colleges. Unfortunately on occasions, tragedies happen and a hypnotherapist may be asked to offer some immediate support to individuals or groups when a student has committed suicide or been murdered.

Animals/pets

People can become very attached to animals/pets, so the loss can be just as great as when losing a human being and therapy may be sought to deal with this. I have used the terms animals and pets, because some clients seeking help may work with animals (e.g. in a cattery, kennel, on a farm); so an animal they lose may not be a pet but one which they have worked with and known for some time. A pet for some people might be the only positive thing or relationship they have in their life.

Relationships

I wanted to put relationships as a separate loss to people and animals/pets. A person can grieve for the actuals relationship rather than a person/animal/pet – what they enjoyed, gained and benefited from the time spent with the person (e.g. companionship; attention; support; experiencing activities/outings; positive feelings).

Objects/possessions

I created this group heading not to talk about material wealth here, but rather to acknowledge that people can keep things for sentimental reasons and losing that object/possession can be devastating. Typical examples being the loss of:

- Anything from a ticket to a concert or a programme from a theatre visit
- Photographs; letters; diaries; writings; poems; cards
- Books; family bible
- Pressed flowers
- Clothes/jewellery (maybe of no monetary value at all).

We all misplace things at some time or other, which can be very annoying, but usually we shall eventually find what we have lost. A totally different situation is if someone steals something from you or a tragedy happens (e.g. possessions lost when there is a house fire or flood).

Some thought must also be given to theft and things being stolen with the intention of doing so. Many different things can be stolen from a person, which are never found or returned. It can be another good exercise to think about everything that has been taken from you through childhood, adolescence and in adulthood. The types of theft a hypnotherapist is likely to deal with in their practice are when any of the following have been stolen from a client:

- Money (e.g. fraudulent activity; burglary; bank account hacked; contested wills)
- Possessions
- Identity
- Ideas (e.g. stolen by a colleague in the workplace and presented as their own initiative to higher management)
- Work produced (e.g. essay; report).

Health/wellbeing

We often take a lot of things for granted – health being a good example. We go about our daily lives and do not think twice about it until we are struck down with a terrible cold or some sort of infection. We then realise how dreadful we feel and how we are unable to do the most simplest of tasks. Physical health is a given for most people, so when it declines or something happens it can seem like a terrible loss, which can then result in further or multiple losses. The importance of mental health has gradually gained more recognition and having a mental health condition is not stigmatised in the same way as it was years ago. Hypnotherapists will be contacted by people who need help with some aspect of their mental health. A person's wellbeing will be affected by both their physical and mental health. The nine aspects of wellbeing as defined in the *Care Act 2014*[7] are as follows:

- Personal dignity (including treatment of the individual with respect)
- Physical and mental health and emotional well-being
- Protection from abuse and harm
- Control by the individual over day-to-day life (including over care and support provided and the way it is provided)
- Participation in work, education, training or recreation
- Social and economic well-being
- Domestic, family and personal relationships
- Suitability of living accommodation
- The individual's contribution to society.

A person could experience some type of loss in relation to any of those aspects of their wellbeing/life.

There are numerous conditions, diseases, illnesses which could affect both physical health and/or mental health. The impact of the Covid-19 pandemic was discussed in Chapter 1. Treatments or surgery could result in losses (e.g. hair after chemotherapy; a limb after amputation). What follows below are some examples of losses a hypnotherapist might have to work with when a client has a problem with their physical or mental health:

- Mobility
- Body part
- Memory/cognitive ability/capacity
- Senses/sensory awareness
- Control
- Dignity, independence, choice.

A hypnotherapist could also work with a client who feels they have 'lost' a person through an illness or disease. A very common example would be the partner of someone who has developed Alzheimer's disease and their personality has changed completely. This situation can also arise when someone is caring for someone with a brain injury or who has suffered a stroke.

Purpose

People who experience a major loss in their life may feel like they have no reason to carry on, that is, they have no purpose. Typically a bereaved person may feel like this and so can a teenager being dumped by the love of their life for the first (but probably not the last) time. Some people might say you cannot compare those two experiences of loss. Making comparisons is not useful because to the person who is experiencing the loss it is probably affecting them greatly. When a major loss is experienced it might feel there is no purpose to life anymore – what is the point? It is important to consider other situations (to look wider than relationships and death) where all meaning and purpose have disappeared and understand why a person may feel they have nothing left or to live for. Attention needs to be given to loss of skills, knowledge, experience, development, opportunities and income through redundancy and retirement. A person can also feel a loss of purpose when they are rejected after a job interview or a younger person cannot get into an education establishment, do the course they want or find a job. A person who is made redundant or forced to take early retirement may also feel purposeless.

Time/stages in life

A person can feel they have lost part of their life because at some point they lost their liberty and maybe their human rights. They may have experienced being locked in somewhere or they have been (or still are) in an institution. Typical examples are:

- Older person having had tuberculosis or polio as a child and being isolated in a hospital for a considerable part of their childhood
- Child or adult experiences of being in hospital for long durations or frequently because of a certain condition requiring regular treatment
- Being sectioned and having to stay in a psychiatric facility

- Being sentenced to a young offenders unit or prison
- Living in: a children's home; a care/nursing home.

For anyone who has been incarcerated in some way and lost their freedom they may have lost their:

- Individuality
- Identity
- Rights
- Privacy
- Respect
- Independence
- Choice
- Dignity
- Fulfilment.

Throughout my social work career I have worked with victims of abuse – both children and adults. Adult survivors have often said to me that they feel they lost their childhood, that is, they never had or experienced what other children did. All victims of abuse are controlled by their perpetrators in some way and lose their freedom to live their lives as they wish to do. Women and men who are living in domestic abuse situations are often coerced and controlled; they are trapped in the situation. The same could be said of anyone who is a victim of a forced marriage or modern slavery.

People who have been in a war can also feel they have lost part of their lives. Writings about the Holocaust and the two world wars can give the hypnotherapist a lot of useful insights into this and is essential if working with an older person who has had these experiences. The works of Judith Hassan are particularly helpful in relation to survivors of the Holocaust.[8] It must be remembered that a hypnotherapist could also work with an asylum seeker/refugee (young or older) who has experienced and seen many atrocities. So in addition to working on trauma it will probably be necessary to work on the related losses e.g. home, family, country, culture etc.

Older people do seek help from hypnotherapists and may need help in facing earlier life experiences and trauma in order to go through the healing process. I use the term 'healing' deliberately because I believe people need to heal and I reject the terminology and any language that suggests that someone is broken and needs to be fixed.

The future

A person who has experienced a loss may need to work on accepting that the future is not as they thought/wanted it to be and they have to plan for a very different future. For a person who has a terminal illness the future may seem very time limited. Whatever the situation, it may seem to the client that they have lost their future. Therefore, it is imperative that the hypnotherapist endeavours to work on the here and now; and encouraging positivity for the time that is left. A large part of the work should be focussed on planning for the immediate future and working on realistic objectives.

Summary of losses

As I said at the beginning of this chapter, the types of losses discussed in the groupings above are not exhaustive. In the following chapter I discuss the importance of assessment and include examples of questionnaires and an exercise which will help the hypnotherapist to work with a client to identify losses. What follows in Appendix 3.1 below is a summary of losses, which can be developed into a handout for use in assessment. The losses are in no particular order of importance and I have included words that have been used by my own clients.

Notes

1 https://dictionary.cambridge.org/dictionary/english/loss.
2 Oxford Compact English Dictionary (2008) Oxford: Oxford University Press.
3 https://www.collinsdictionary.com/dictionary/english/loss.
4 https://www.merriam-webster.com/dictionary/loss.
5 https://www.thefreedictionary.com/loss.
6 National Crime Agency (24th March 2021) UK Missing Persons Unit. *Missing Persons Report 2019/20*, https://www.nationalcrimeagency.gov.uk/who-we-are/publications/501-uk-missing-persons-unit-data-report-2019-2020/file.
7 *Care Act 2014*, https://www.legislation.gov.uk/ukpga/2014/23/contents/enacted.
8 Hassan, J. (2013) 'Recovery and healing in the survivors of the holocaust'. In J. Pritchard (ed) *Good Practice in Promoting Recovery and Healing for Abused Adults'* London: Jessica Kingsley Publishers.
   Hassan, J. (2003) *A House Next Door to Trauma: Learning from Holocaust Survivors How to Respond to Atrocity*. London: Jessica Kingsley Publishers.

Appendix 3.1: Summary of different types of losses

- People
- Pets
- Relationships
- Objects
- Health
- Wellbeing
- Physical health
- Mental health
- Ability
- Capacity
- Memory
- Purpose
- Direction
- Stages of life
- Time/years
- Freedom
- Human rights
- Hope
- Ambition/aspirations
- Future
- Privacy
- Independence
- Individuality
- Identity
- Dignity
- Choice
- Fulfilment
- Respect
- Confidence/self esteem
- Values
- Trust
- Faith/belief
- Control
- Power
- Decision making
- Employment
- Income/money
- Wealth/assets
- Opportunity
- Experience
- Knowledge
- Skills
- Safety/security
- Love
- Affection
- Attention
- Friendship
- Companionship.

4 Assessment before working with losses

A properly trained hypnotherapist will understand the importance of assessment and should allocate enough time to assess a client before introducing them to hypnosis and developing a treatment plan. However, hypnotherapists will have their own preference regarding how they will undertake their assessments. For example, some hypnotherapists advertise on their websites that they offer a free 15 or 30 minute consultation on the phone. Since the onset of the Covid-19 pandemic more hypnotherapists offer services online/remotely (e.g. using Zoom, Skype or Facetime) and as such will assess in this way. In my own practice I prefer to do the assessment face-to-face and be able to observe the client's body language whilst we are talking. When working remotely it is not always possible to closely observe a client's body language as only their top half may be visible. Observing breathing patterns is also very important and again this can sometimes be hindered when working remotely. I will always talk to a potential client on the telephone and this can be at length, but it is not what I call a proper assessment – rather information gathering. During that telephone conversation I will glean information about the potential client and the reason for seeking help and I will talk about:

- Hypnosis: what it is and what it is not
- My own particular way of working
- What I can offer (individual/group sessions)
- Consent and confidentiality
- Notes and record keeping
- Assessment in a first session.

Even if I have spent half an hour talking on the phone with a potential client, I will undertake a thorough assessment during their first appointment. This can take between 30 and 45 minutes and is free of charge.

No matter how a hypnotherapist is going to undertake their assessments, the objective should be to obtain information about the following

DOI: 10.4324/9781032245706-5

subjects – some of which will not be relevant to all clients but still have to be checked out:

- Personal details
- Contact details
- Significant people in personal/work life; friends; family; colleagues
- Any professionals/workers involved
- Physical health: current and past
- Mental health: current and past
- Medication/treatment/surgery
- Any current issues/problems (in addition to the presenting problem)
- Counselling/therapy: current and/or previous
- Hypnosis: knowledge/understanding/previous experience
- Fears/phobias
- Hobbies/interests
- Reason for attending for hypnotherapy/objectives/wishes.

Assessment when dealing with loss or bereavement

I have discussed previously that a loss may only be identified once hypnotherapy has started; this could even be after a couple of sessions have taken place. However, there are times when a person will make contact to specifically ask for help with a particular loss or bereavement; or a person is terminally ill and wants help with facing and planning for their death. I have developed a specific questionnaire for these referrals/situations (which can also be used when a loss is identified after hypnotherapy has started), which is presented in Appendix 4.1. The questionnaire can be used in the conscious state or in the trance state. It includes questions for general assessment (covering subject areas as listed above) and then for more specific subject areas (the hypnotherapist will utilise as appropriate):

1 General assessment

Have you seen a hypnotherapist before? (If yes, how was that experience? Was anything particularly helpful or unhelpful?)
How much do you know about hypnosis?
How would you describe your general state of health?
Have you ever had an operation? (If yes, please state when and what for)
Are you currently taking any medication? (If yes, please give details)
Do you have any diagnosed medical conditions? (If yes, please give details)
Do you have epilepsy or narcolepsy?
Do you ever experience any breathing difficulties e.g. asthma; hay fever? (If yes, do you use an inhaler?)

Have you ever been referred to a psychiatrist? (If yes, for what reason?)
Have you any fears or phobias?
What are your interests/hobbies?

2 Dealing with a loss(es)

What loss have you experienced?
What loss are you dealing with now?
What loss do you want to work on/deal with?
When did the loss happen?
How has the loss affected you personally?
How has the loss affected your life in general?
Has the loss affected anyone else?
How did the loss affect you at the time?
How is it affecting you now?
On a scale of 1 to 10 how is it adversely affecting your life? (Scale: 1 = little effect; 10 = greatly affected)
What do you want to change?
What do you want to be different?

3 Bereavement

Who has died?
When did this happen (get exact date if possible)?
What happened?
Was it expected or sudden?
Have you been bereaved before? If yes, who have you lost?
Were you present at the death?
How did you feel at the time?
How has the death affected you?
How do you feel now?
What do you feel you need help with?
On a scale of 1 to 10 how is it affecting your life? (Scale: 1 = little effect; 10 = greatly affected)
Do you know anything about the stages of grief?

4 Terminal illness

Tell me about your illness.
What has your doctor said to you about your future?
How are you feeling about being terminally ill/dying/death?
What emotions have you felt already?
What are you feeling now?
Do you have any particular worries/concerns/fears?
What do you want to work on?

What would you like to discuss?
Are there things you need to do?
What do you want to plan for?
Has anyone close to you died?
Have you seen anyone die?
Do you believe there is something after this life?
Is there any other information you think might be helpful for me to know?

An exercise for identifying losses

People are often more resilient than they think they are; and I think this is a very important point to remember when thinking about losses experienced in life. A person will probably remember major losses which have occurred in their life but what might be referred to as simple day-to-day losses may not be remembered at all (although they will be embedded in the subconscious mind somewhere). The subconscious mind is there to protect a person. It will do what it thinks is in a person's best interests. It can suppress memories because it deems that is the best way to protect someone. It can be much easier to remember things when in the trance state.

Losses may be identified when working with a client on an issue and then worked on because they are recognised as the root cause of the problem. Some hypnotherapists use regression techniques to work on the past rather than adopting the solution-focussed approach. However, a hypnotherapist when undertaking an assessment can become aware that there has been a series of losses in a client's life which s/he is not linking up at all. Another circumstance can be that a client presents for help with a loss, grief or bereavement and then other losses come to the forefront. I developed the following exercise, which can be used either in the conscious state or in the trance state. A form is included in Appendix 4.2 which can be used by the hypnotherapist; or it can be given to the client to do during the hypnotherapy session or as a piece of homework to do between sessions. It is a useful exercise to use during an assessment and can be revisited in future sessions when more losses may be identified. Once a client starts thinking about losses – more may be acknowledged.

Script for exercise

I do not want you to try too hard with this – just go with your gut initially. The purpose of the exercise is to get you to think about different types of losses you have experienced.

1 Recent losses

Think back over the past week. What losses have you experienced?

Now think back over the past month. What losses have you experienced?
(Guidance note: the hypnotherapist repeats the question for the following time periods)

Past 3 months
Past 6 months
Up to 12 months

2 *Other losses you remember*

(Guidance note: the hypnotherapist should work through the following years/decades with the client using the same question: What losses have you experienced?)

1–2 years
2 –5 years
Last 10 years
Other times in your life (as appropriate: 20/30/40/50 years)
Childhood
Adolescence
Adulthood

What do you consider to have been major losses you have experienced?
What do you consider to have been significant losses you have experienced?
What seemed to be significant losses at the time but now you consider them to be minor or insignificant?
How did this loss affect you?
How did you feel at the time you lost *(insert loss)?*
How do you feel about it now?
What did you learn from experiencing that loss?

Significant dates

During an assessment or when therapy is underway, significant dates can come to light. For example, a client who has miscarried will remember the date of the miscarriage but may also remember the date the baby was due. Some clients will remember specific dates when things actually happened. Others will know their behaviour or feelings change (e.g. they are low/sad; they become short-tempered) at a certain time of year and yet they do not know why. The hypnotherapist who uses regression may explore this and find the reason for the changes, and possibly the exact significant date or time something happened. For these situations and for the hypnotherapist to keep a written record, I have included in Appendix 4.3 a form for significant dates. In some cases, the client may wish to commemorate the date in some way e.g. when the date is the anniversary of a happy event or of a death and they wish to celebrate the life of the person who has passed (see Chapter 28).

Self-analysis for hypnotherapists

I think it is also important to consider self-analysis for hypnotherapists whilst talking about assessment and working with losses. Any therapist needs to self-reflect regularly for their own personal and professional development. It is imperative that a therapist works on their own issues. Supervision sessions are a good place to do this or if it is a specialist issue then the right resource/help should be sought. When training to become a hypnotherapist, some reflection and work should have been undertaken regarding:

- Personal history
- Unresolved personal issues which need to be addressed before becoming a qualified practitioner
- Any past or current work issues which need addressing
- Life experience: what may be useful when working with clients
- Other work/career experience: which may be transferable and prove useful in the future when practising as a hypnotherapist.

The exercise described above can also prove useful for a hypnotherapist to undertake themselves or during a supervision session in order to explore their losses. I also think that during initial training beliefs, values and attitudes regarding the following subjects should be explored (or if this was not done then it is helpful to think about and discuss them now):

- Death (e.g. any particular fears/bad experiences?)
- Own mortality
- Life after death (e.g. does it exist? If so, in what form?)
- Spirituality.

Appendix 4.1: Questionnaire for general assessment/ loss/ bereavement/terminal illness

Strictly Confidential

QUESTIONNAIRE FOR GENERAL ASSESSMENT/ LOSS/BEREAVEMENT/TERMINAL ILLNESS

Name: Date of Birth:

Address:

Telephone/mobile:

E-mail address:

Significant people (family/friends):

Any professionals involved:

Reason for referral (e.g. type of loss):

1 General assessment

Have you seen a hypnotherapist before? (If yes, how was that experience? Was anything particularly helpful or unhelpful?)

How much do you know about hypnosis?

How would you describe your general state of health?

Have you ever had an operation? (If yes, please state when and what for)

Are you currently taking any medication? (If yes, please give details)

Do you have any diagnosed medical conditions? (If yes, please give details)

Do you have epilepsy or narcolepsy?

Do you ever experience any breathing difficulties e.g. asthma; hay fever? (If yes, do you use an inhaler?)

Have you ever been referred to a psychiatrist? (If yes, for what reason?)

Have you any fears or phobias?

What are your interests/hobbies?

2 *Dealing with a loss(es)*

What loss have you experienced?

What loss are you dealing with now?

What loss do you want to work on/deal with?

When did the loss happen?

How has the loss affected you personally?

How has the loss affected your life in general?

Has the loss affected anyone else?

How did the loss affect you at the time?

How is it affecting you now?

On a scale of 1 to 10 how is it adversely affecting your life? (Scale: 1 = little effect; 10 = greatly affected)

What do you want to change?

What do you want to be different?

3 *Bereavement*

Who has died?

When did this happen (get exact date if possible)?

What happened?

Was it expected or sudden?

Have you been bereaved before? If yes, who have you lost?

Were you present at the death?

How did you feel at the time?

How has the death affected you?

How do you feel now?

What do you feel you need help with?

On a scale of 1 to 10 how is it affecting your life? (Scale: 1 = little effect: 10 = greatly affected)

Do you know anything about the stages of grief?

4 *Terminal illness*

Tell me about your illness.

What has your doctor said to you about your future?

How are you feeling about being terminally ill/dying/death?

What emotions have you felt already?

What are you feeling now?

Do you have any particular worries/concerns/fears?

What do you want to work on?

What would you like to discuss?

Are there things you need to do?

What do you want to plan for?

Has anyone close to you died?

Have you seen anyone die?

Do you believe there is something after this life?

Is there any other information you think might be helpful for me to know?

Appendix 4.2: Form for exercise – identifying losses

IDENTIFYING LOSSES

Name of client: Date exercise undertaken:

Loss   *Detail/information*

1 week

1 month

6 months

12 months

Last 1–2 years

Last 2–5 years

Last 10 years

Last 20/30/30/40/50 years

Childhood

Adolescence

Adulthood

Appendix 4.3: Form for significant dates

SIGNIFICANT DATES

This form can be used to highlight dates, times experiences which need to be worked on or for commemoration purposes.

Date/month/year	*Loss experienced*	*Action needed*
1.		
2.		
3.		
4.		
5.		
6.		
7.		
8.		
9.		
10.		

5 Two scripts for the first session

Introducing hypnosis to the client

Established hypnotherapists will already have numerous ways of demonstrating hypnosis to a client in the first session and will also have an abundance of techniques to get them into the trance state. All of these skills and tools can be utilised when working with a client who comes to deal with a loss. However, I felt it was necessary to put in two introductory scripts for readers who are students or newly qualified hypnotherapists. It is usual to refer to a 'safe place' when working with a client, but when a client has come specifically to work on a loss then I refer to a 'peaceful place', which is the terminology used in script 1. The script also introduces the client to the concept of the journey of grief.

Script 2 uses a magic carpet to introduce the client to the idea that their subconscious mind is a powerful tool. The magic carpet (subconscious mind) can take them anywhere they want to go and embeds the idea of being in control. This is a good script to record for the client so they can practise self-hypnosis before the second session.

Script 1: An introduction to trance

Close your eyes and let go of whatever is going through your mind at this moment in time. To do this it can be helpful to concentrate on your breathing – slowing it down – breathing in very gently – and then breathing out even more gently. You will learn how to control your breathing by breathing in slowly and gently – not gulping – rather breathing in very gently and smoothly. Let's try that now. I am going to use the count of 3. I shall ask you breathe in for 3 and then to hold your breath briefly. Then I shall ask you to let go and breathe out slowly, gently and smoothly for 3.

Breathe in: *1, 2, 3* – and hold
Breathe out: *3, 2, 1* – relax.
Good nice and slow – breathing gently and smoothly. Let's try that again.

DOI: 10.4324/9781032245706-6

Breathe in: *1, 2, 3* – and hold
Breathe out: *3, 2, 1* – relax.
And again.
Breathe in: *1, 2, 3* – and hold
Breathe out: *3, 2, 1* – relax.

You are relaxing more and more now with each breath that you take. So now I am going to ask you to imagine certain things – you may see or sense what I suggest – or your mind might drift somewhere else – and that is fine. Imagine that you are sitting in a very soft, comfortable armchair. So comfortable in fact, you feel as though you are sinking deep down into the chair – and as you do so you are becoming more and more relaxed. In front of you is a fireplace which has a mantelpiece. On the mantelpiece piece there are ten candles – all alight – and flickering away. You may feel some warmth coming from the candles which is very soothing and comforting. At the same time the warmth is relaxing you more and more – as you continue to breathe slowly, gently and smoothly. Keep looking at the candles. Look at the size of each candle – look at the colour or colours you can see. The flickering flames are relaxing you more and more.

In a moment I am going to count down from *10* down to *1*. As you hear me say a number, the flame on one of the candles will go out and a part of your body will relax.

10: A candle goes out. Your head tilts and relaxes
9: Another candle goes out. All your face relaxes – your muscles – your forehead – your cheekbones – your mouth – your jaw and your teeth. The candles keep going out each time you hear another number
8: Your neck and throat relax – feel comfortable
7: Your right arm relaxes – down to your hand, fingers and thumb
6: Your left arm relaxes – down to your hand, fingers and thumb
5: Your spine sinks further into the back of the soft, comfortable armchair. All the muscles around your spine become floppy and relaxed. The flames continue to go out.
4: Your chest and stomach relax. Sinking deeper and deeper into the soft, comfortable armchair.
3: Your right leg relaxes – down to your feet and toes
2: Your left leg relaxes – down to your feet and toes
1: Now all the flames are out. The room is dark. Your body is completely relaxed – your mind is completely relaxed.

Somewhere in the room where you are sitting there is a door. Look around the room and you will see where the door is because there will be some faint light coming into the room from underneath the door. When you see where the door is, get up out of the soft, comfortable armchair and walk towards the door. In a moment you are going to open the door and go out of the room. When you come out of the room you will find yourself in a place where you feel totally at peace with yourself and at peace with the world. This will be your peaceful place. On the count of *3* – open the door – *1, 2*, and *3* – now walk out of the room and find your peaceful place. You feel at peace with yourself and at peace with the world. Walk around now – explore your peaceful place.

(Guidance note: if working in a group the hypnotherapist should leave a few minutes for clients to explore the peaceful place before continuing with the prompts below. If working with one client, specific direct questions can be asked)

I wonder:

- What you are seeing in your peaceful place
- If you are hearing anything
- If you are smelling anything
- If you can taste anything in your mouth
- If you want to change anything
- If you want to bring anything into your peaceful place
- How you are feeling.

Coming to meet with me here today means that you have already started your journey of grief and you are now ready to continue the journey. The journey may not be easy. At times you will see the road ahead clearly – at other times the road might be in darkness – or in a mist or fog. It will not always be an easy journey – you have a lot to face. There will be bumps in the road. You might have to take a detour and end up in a place you did not expect. At times the journey could be hard going. You will sometimes feel tired from travelling, but you can always take a rest. It does not matter how you travel. You will travel in a way that is right for you. It does not matter how long it takes you to complete the journey. You will travel at a pace that suits you. You can take all the time you need. You will find exciting, new places to explore. You will really enjoy parts of the journey as you learn about you as a traveller as well as other people and places on the way. One thing I know for sure is that you will complete your journey – you will do it in your own time – you will get there – to your final destination. You will reach your final destination – the end of your journey of grief – in your own time.

Script 2: Magic carpet

Imagine that you are in a very large, spacious carpet shop. Take a look around you. You will see that there are so many rolls of carpet. Some are standing upright on the floor – others are leaning against the wall and some are wrapped around big rollers hanging off the walls. There are so many different carpets – so many different materials – textures – colours. Even though the shop has so many carpets you feel a sense of space – as though you can walk around and not be restricted – a sense you can go anywhere you want. So start walking around.

As you start walking around the carpet shop and looking at all the different rolls of carpet I wonder if you might like to touch the carpets – see what they are made of – feel the textures – look deep into the colours. Some carpets will be all one colour – look for the different shades of dark and light. Other carpets will have lots of colours – look for any patterns you can see. I wonder if you can smell anything as you walk by the carpets.

You become aware of other things nearby – small pieces of carpet cut off from the larger rolls – carpet tiles – mats and rugs. You are aware again of the different materials – textures – colours. Go and touch the carpets – carpet tiles – mats and rugs if you want to do so.

In one corner you see a pile of carpets. There is a notice above the pile of carpets which says: 'Magic Carpets'. I wonder how curious you are. It can be good to explore and find new things. Do you want to find out more? I wonder if you are curious to find out what a magic carpet can do – where a magic carpet can take you. I wonder how magical the carpets are – how powerful they are.

Now walk over to the pile of magic carpets. Have a good look at them. Touch them – move them – take some out from the pile and take a closer look. See which ones you like. Somewhere in that pile there is a magic carpet that has been made just for you – it is exactly right for you. Keep looking for it – you will know when you see it. Tell me when you have found it.

*(Guidance note: if working with an individual the hypnotherapist can ask
the client to describe their magic carpet)*

Now sit on your magic carpet. You are feeling excited – excited about going on a journey. You can go anywhere you want to go. Your magic carpet is there for you – it can take you in any direction you want to travel. You can tell it where you want to go – which direction you want to take. Or maybe you will just let your magic carpet surprise you – let it take you somewhere it knows you need to visit.

So when you are ready tell your magic carpet to lift off the floor. Tell it to start flying around the shop. You are in control. You can tell your magic carpet to fly high – going up and up – going higher and higher. You can tell it to fly lower – going down and down – getting lower and lower. You can control the speed of your magic carpet too – you can make it go faster or slower. Alter the speed now – go faster – then go slower. Try out your magic carpet – turning it to the right – turning it to the left. I wonder if it can turn upside down or spin around. Your magic carpet can do all sorts of things. So have some fun travelling around the carpet shop – experiment with your magic carpet – see what it can do.

(Guidance note: if working with an individual the hypnotherapist can ask the client to explain what the magic carpet is doing. If working with a group, sufficient time should be left for experimentation – this should not rushed)

Now it is time to broaden your horizons. Explore new places. So when you are ready your magic carpet will take you towards the entrance doors of the shop – the doors will open – out you go into the big wide world – full of places and things to experience – people to meet – new opportunities. So out you go – through the doors – up and up towards the sky. See again what your magic carpet can do. Remember you are in control. Tell your magic carpet to fly high – going up and up – going higher and higher. Tell your magic carpet to fly lower – going down and down – getting lower and lower. Now alter the speed of your magic carpet – make it go faster or slower. Try it now – go faster – then go slower. Do whatever you want – you are in control.

So enjoy the journey now – go wherever you would like to go or just let your magic carpet take you to where you need to be.

(Guidance note: in future sessions the magic carpet can be used to go forward in time to forward pace or back in time as a regression technique)

Part II
Dealing with emotions

6 Journey of grief

Grief is often seen as a negative thing but in fact grieving is a very positive process. People need to grieve in order to face a loss, work through it and eventually accept it. The timing and duration of the process will differ for each person. It can be helpful to think of grief as a journey and I adopt this approach when working with losses and bereavement. So this theme and term 'journey of grief' is used throughout this book. I would recommend that a hypnotherapist who is going to work with losses and bereavement should read the established and extensive works of both Elizabeth Kubler-Ross[1] and Colin Murray Parkes.[2] In her early work Kubler-Ross was focussing very much on how people/professionals can help with death and dying. In 2004 she said 'There is no correct way or time to grieve' (Kubler-Ross and Kessler, p. xvii[3]). I think it is so important for any professional to keep reminding themselves of this. We are living in an era where it so common for people to say: 'Move on' or 'It's time you moved on'. This is not helpful when someone is still working their way through a loss and grieving.

Kubler-Ross did develop a model of the stages of grief in 1969, which has been referred to worldwide over decades. The five stages are:

1 Denial
2 Anger
3 Bargaining
4 Depression
5 Acceptance.

She explains in her original work that the five stages are:

> ...part of the framework that makes up our learning to live with the one we lost. They are tools to help us frame and identify what we may be feeling. But they are not stops on some linear timeline in grief. Not everyone goes through all of them or goes in a prescribed order.

> (*On Death and Dying*, 1969, p.7)

DOI: 10.4324/9781032245706-8

Parkes[4] similarly developed a model of grief which has four stages:

1   Shock and numbness
2   Yearning and searching
3   Disorganisation and despair
4   Reorganisation and recovery.

As already stated above, in this book I shall refer to the journey of grief, which will be for any type of loss – not just death and bereavement. The term is used in many of the scripts. The departure point is the loss of a person, animal, relationship, object or situation. The destination is living a new way of life, having accepted the loss and adjusted to the changes that have occurred as a result of that loss.

The hypnotherapist can work with the subconscious mind to take the grieving person on all sorts of journeys to deal with their thoughts, feelings and behaviours. Some may prefer to use longer scripts to achieve this. However, it can be useful to use individual visualisations to help the client realise that things can be changed and the journey of grief will come to an end. What follows are some visualisations for this purpose. The client needs to understand that the journey of grief will not be smooth; they will need to face and work through many emotions. The visualisations address some of the difficulties/feelings the client may have to face on their own journey of grief. I find it helpful to use a visualisation in the first session when introducing the concept of the journey of grief to the client; and then to repeat or use other visualisations in future sessions. Other visualisations to deal specifically with emotional pain are presented Chapter 9.

1 Steep hill to climb

Some people will tell you that 'time is a great healer'; others might say 'it's time to move on'. They do not mean to be unkind but sometimes their words do not help. Not when you are feeling tired – lethargic – worn out – worn down – that you have little or no energy at all – that you have little or no motivation. It can help to imagine certain things so you can acknowledge that life will get better – when the time is right for you – you do not have to rush things.

Imagine that you are going to take a walk up a hill. This hill is situated in a very beautiful area. If you look around you can see lots of trees, bushes, grass and flowers. Nobody else is about – just you and the sounds of nature.

Before you start walking, look at the hill in front of you. You see that it is quite steep. You might feel like you just do not have the energy to walk up it. Even though you know it will be good exercise for you and there will be a beautiful view when you reach the top of the hill. You see a road that you can walk on. This road will take you to the top of the hill and then you can go down the other side and you will see new things. It will be worth the climb. Just think about it. You can climb that hill – even if you are feeling tired – lethargic – worn out – worn down – that you have little or no energy at all. But you know don't you – if you do climb the hill, you will feel better once you reach the top and see new things on the other side? Leaving all your tiredness behind you.

Take some deep breaths – you know you can do this – look at the hill – and now start walking. Just go at a steady pace. I know you have been feeling tired – lethargic – worn out – worn down – that you have little or no energy at all. But that is changing. You want to do this – climb the hill – and see the view on the other side. You can do this and you will do this, won't you? Stretch your legs out – walk at a steady pace. Breathe in and then breathe out – in and out. Just take it steady. Start to walk away from the tiredness – the lethargy – everything that has been making you feel terrible *(insert anything specific the client has talked about)*. You can build your strength in your body and in your mind as you walk up the hill. So keep walking.

Up and up the hill you go. Feeling stronger with each step. Keep going. Feeling determined to reach the top. Feeling energised with each step. Feel your calf muscles strengthening with each step. Feel your arms swinging freely. Feel your head getting lighter. Keep walking up the hill. Feeling stronger with each step. Keep going. Feeling energised with each step. You want to see the other side of the hill. You want to see and experience new things. Things will be different on the other side. You start to feel excited about how different the view will be on the other side of the hill. Keep going. Up and up the hill. Higher and higher. Feeling good – feeling strong – feeling energised – feeling excited – feeling lighter.

You are nearly at the top of the hill now. You feel so much better. You cannot wait now to get to the top of the hill and see the view on the other side. You notice you are walking faster and faster now because you want to get there – you want to see the view – the other side of the hill where the new things are. And then you are there. Look at the view. Look at the new things. Look at what is in front of you.

2 A bumpy ride

Imagine that you are on a small rowing boat, but somehow the boat has got lost and has ended up in the ocean. You are sitting in the boat, which is rocking from side to side. You look out across the ocean. You see waves coming towards the boat. They are fairly large in size and moving rapidly. The boat rocks from side to side very quickly. You start to feel sick. You think you might actually be sick. You grab both sides of the boat to try and steady yourself. One big wave suddenly rushes over you and the boat. You are drenched with water – soaked through – your hair – your clothes – your shoes. You see another big wave coming and you feel a wave of sickness again, but you also feel a sense of panic. You feel out of control. The boat rocks faster and faster – from side to side – and then another wave goes over you and the boat. The water rushes all over you. You feel swamped and out of control. You do not know what to do. It is all too much – a little boat in the big ocean.

You need to take control of the boat. Even though it might be small in size the boat has been well built. It is strong and sturdy. It has been built with good quality wood by people who understand that art of building a boat to make it safe to travel in. You know it can weather any storm – rough seas – big waves. The boat needs to go with the waves. Ride up and down on the waves – go with the waves. So, you need to go with the boat and the waves too.

While the boat rides the waves up and down – up and down up – it is OK for you to experience different emotions. You know these feelings will not last forever. You just have to ride the waves. So if you feel sick – that is OK. If you are sick that is OK too. If you feel lost – that is OK. If you feel panicky – that is OK. If you feel swamped that is OK. If you feel like you are sinking that is OK *(insert any other feeling/emotion the client may have talked about)*. When you feel any of these emotions you will know they will not last forever, so you can stay with those feelings and then work through them. Then they will be gone. The waves will stop going up and down – and eventually the ocean will become flat – calm.

So do that now. Ride the waves – up and down. Experience those different feelings – one at a time. Stay with a feeling and work through it. Sick. Lost. Panicky. Swamped *(and anything else relevant to the client)*. As you experience and work through a feeling the waves become smaller – the boat rocks less and less. The waves become smaller – the boat rocks less and less. Watch how the waves become smaller and smaller – the ocean becomes calmer and calmer – you feel calmer and calmer. The waves become smaller and smaller – the ocean becomes calmer and calmer – you feel calmer and calmer. The waves have gone – the ocean is flat and calm.

3 Valley of despair

Imagine you see in the distance a valley – a very deep valley. On either side of the valley you see huge mountains. The mountains are extremely high so the drop into the valley is very steep. Getting down into the valley can be gradual or it can happen very quickly. It depends what is happening on the mountains and around them – what the conditions are. The weather. The soil on the ground. The rocks.

Imagine now that you are standing on top of one of the mountains. Look down into the deep valley. I wonder whether you can actually see all the way down there – maybe it is too far into the distance. Everything seems a bit blurry. Now I want you to imagine that you have the ability to fly, because you are going to fly down – down into the deep valley. Before you do that I want you to focus on how you have been feeling lately. You have talked about feeling in despair *(insert any other words the client may have used describing/relating to despair)* – as though there is no hope – no future. As you fly down into the valley you will experience those feelings again. Get ready now to fly off the top of the mountain. Ready – steady – and off you go. Fly down into the deep valley.

You are flying down and down and down – feel that despair – feel that sinking feeling – sinking down and down and down. Maybe feeling out of control as you swerve in your descent towards the valley. Swaying off to the right and then swaying off to the left. Out of control – feeling as though you are sinking – being pulled in all different directions before you sink further down and down and down. You are flying faster and faster as you descend into the valley. You do not feel as though you can stop. You may feel scared because you cannot stop these feelings – but you can stop them – and you will stop them.

Keep flying down – you start to see the valley a little more clearly. It looks dark down there. You cannot see any grass or any other greenery. It looks very bare in the valley. You are getting closer and closer now. Suddenly you land with a huge thud – totally unexpected. You are in the valley.

The valley is very dark – you find it hard to see anything. You look around you – surrounded by darkness. You also feel cold – and start to shiver. You feel lost because you cannot see any way out of the valley. It is dark and gloomy. The ground underneath your feet is very hard and rocky – making it difficult to walk. You try to walk forward but you stumble and lose your balance. You just cannot see which way to go. You may feel as if you will never get out of the valley.

You are a resourceful person. You need to make a fire to create some light so you can see the way forward. Start looking around you. At first you might not see what you need – things can be hidden. There will be things in this valley that can be used to make a fire – a fire which will burn brightly so you can see the way out of the valley. Find what you need to make the fire. Now start to make the fire and light it. Watch the fire start to burn – small flames growing into bigger flames. The flames are making it brighter – the darkness is fading. It is getting brighter and brighter. You can see around you now. Everything becomes brighter and clearer. You can see very clearly now. You can see the way out of the deep valley. You see the huge mountains on either side. You know which way to go now. You are ready to go. So make your way out of the deep valley.

4 Erupting like a volcano

Feeling angry has a purpose – it does not necessarily have to be a negative thing. Obviously it would be negative if the anger resulted in someone being harmed. Anger is an emotion and it can serve a purpose. Your subconscious mind wants you to experience anger for a reason. Your subconscious mind is always working for your benefit. I know you have been feeling very angry because you have lost *(insert the loss)*. Sometimes you may feel that you do not know what to do with this anger, so it can be helpful to imagine certain things to get rid of the feeling.

Imagine that you have travelled to an unfamiliar place, and in front of you there is what looks like a huge black mountain. The mountain is black because it is covered in dark rocks. What you are actually looking at is a volcano. The rocks have been made from lava which has previously erupted out of the volcano. As you are standing there you feel that your feet are starting to feel very warm. Just concentrate on feeling your feet. They are getting warmer and warmer. Bend down and touch the ground with one of your hands – you will feel that the ground is very warm. Leave your hand on the ground and feel the temperature increase. The ground – your hand – and both your feet – are getting warmer and warmer.

Stand up again. Feel the warmth rising up from the ground – into your feet – and feel it go up your legs. You are starting to feel uncomfortable because you now feel hot not just warm. The heat continues to travel up your body. The heat is like your anger – it rises – it expands – it goes in different directions. It makes you feel uncomfortable. You might feel irritable – short tempered. You want to stop the heat rising just like you want to stop feeling angry. But the heat just carries on – becoming stronger and stronger.

Now look at the volcano again. You can see smoke rising from rocks that have already formed on the volcano. The smoke is rising up and up into the air – reaching towards the sky. Look now to the very top of the volcano – the crater – you see thick lava rising from the summit of the volcano. It is thick and spiralling upwards. Just like the anger you feel. I wonder where your anger starts – in your stomach – or your head – or somewhere else. Wherever it starts it spirals like the smoke out of the volcano. Thick dark lava – you cannot see through it – you cannot see a way to stop the lava spiralling and spreading. Sometimes you just have to wait – experience what is happening – it is happening for a reason.

Keep watching the lava rising from the crater – rising from the top of the volcano. The lava is getting thicker and thicker – rising higher and higher. You feel more and more uncomfortable – angry. Watch the lava coming out of the crater. Look more closely to the edge of the crater – you see some different colours – orange and red. The molten rock in the volcano starts off a very bright orange colour, then it turns red and when the lava gets out into the open it turns black.

The volcano is getting very hot inside now. Lots of bright orange molten rock is bubbling deep within the volcano. Getting hotter and hotter – brighter and brighter – hotter and hotter. The volcano is getting ready to erupt. You are waiting for the volcano to erupt. *1, 2,* and *3* and bang – the volcano erupts.

And suddenly you feel a sense of release – a sense of freedom. You are cooling down. You start to feel comfortable. You are getting cooler and cooler – more comfortable – calm – calmer and calmer. You feel comfortable as the lava rolls down the sides of the volcano – settling on the sides of the volcano. Cooler and cooler – calmer and calmer. The lava is turning to rock as it cools down. The fire is out.

Anytime in the future when you feel anger rising within you, just think of the volcano and watch it. Wait for the eruption and then you will feel cool, comfortable and calm – at peace with yourself.

5 Avoiding the puddles

You are standing on a pavement. It has been raining heavily for hours and hours, so a lot of very deep puddles have formed on the pavement. It continues to rain. Look in front of you and count how many puddles you can see along the pavement. As you count, the rain continues to fall. It seems endless. Rain – rain – and more rain. Falling down – down – and down. Keep counting the puddles.

You feel miserable standing in the rain. You could start walking and find somewhere to shelter, but something is not letting you do that. I wonder what is stopping you from finding shelter. I wonder why you sometimes make things harder for yourself. You know that you need to face some things – some facts – some situations – or some people – in order to make things better. You are still standing in the rain. You feel like you are rooted to the spot. You do not want to move forward – even though you are feeling cold, wet and alone. Look at the puddles again. They seem to have expanded and multiplied. In parts it is hard to see the pavement at all.

So brace yourself. You are going to walk along the pavement – you are going to get out of the rain. On the count of three start walking – *1, 2, and 3*. I wonder which way you are walking. Are you trying to avoid the puddles? If you are – think about the reason for avoiding the puddles. Sometimes you need to go straight forward and if that means going through a puddle – walking right to it and then through the middle of it – and getting wet – then do it.

Throughout life everyone has to do things they do not want to do and face things they do not want to face. It can be easier to avoid things – go into denial – but nothing will be resolved until you deal with things head on. Just like the puddles in front of you. They are expanding on the pavement and getting deeper. You are going to have to go through some of them. It may feel that things are getting worse – that you are sinking lower and lower – and to face reality is just not something you want to do. But to get to warmth and safety you need to face things. So deal with those puddles now.

Keep walking and walk through the puddles. Think about what you need to deal with – what or who you need to face. See whatever you are thinking about in the puddle in front of you. You need to deal with and get through the puddle in front of you. Step into it now. Go further in. Find out how deep it is. Look down into the puddle – I wonder what you are seeing and feeling now. You can get through this puddle. It is time to continue – take a step out of the puddle. That was not too bad was it?

Keep walking. Walk through another puddle – this one is even deeper. You sink in the rainwater – right up to your ankles. Your feet and ankles are really wet now – so you might as well splash about in the puddle a bit. Find out how deep the puddle is. What else can you find in the puddle? Is there some rubbish – a takeaway tray – sweet wrappers – a pop can or bottle – I do not know what might be there, but you can find out. Explore. Now kick out the rubbish from the puddle to make your way out clear. You can get through this puddle. It is time to continue – take a step out of the puddle. That was not too bad was it?

Now find another puddle. You are feeling more confident now that you can walk through puddles. You do not have to avoid them. You can deal with whatever you find in a puddle and then step out. I wonder what you will find in the next puddle. Have some fun – explore – splash about – stamp about – do whatever feels right. Feel confident that you can face anything or anyone. You can make your way through any puddle – shallow or deep – you can face and deal with anything or anyone or any situation in the future.

Notes

1 Elizabeth Kubler-Ross' original work *On Death and Dying* was written back in the 1969 and there have been many anniversary editions produced since then. It is worth reading a version. She wrote many other books too; all of which will enrich a hypnotherapist's knowledge and understanding of death and dying, but also regarding grief and grieving.
2 Colin Murray Parkes, like Kubler-Ross, has written extensively over the years and I would recommend in particular reading one of his older texts: Parkes, C. M. and Markus, A. (1998) *Coping with Loss.* London: BMJ Books.
3 Kubler-Ross, E. and Kessler, D. (2014) *On Grief and Grieving: Finding the Meaning of Grief Through the Five Stages of Loss.* London: Simon and Schuster Inc.
4 Parkes, C.M. and Prigerson, H.G. (2010) *Bereavement: Studies of Grief in Adult Life* 4th Edition. London: Penguin.

7   Tour bus

Introduction

The script was originally written in order to introduce the concept of the journey of grief in a first session. However, in my own practice over the years I have found it more useful to use shorter visualisations (as presented in the previous chapter) in a first session and then introduce the tour bus in the second session. It can then be revisited in future sessions as the client travels on their journey of grief. The client is initially taken on a tour in order to realise that there will be many things to see and experience on the journey but there may also be obstacles and detours along the way.

There is a tour guide on the bus (i.e. the subconscious mind), which is written as a male in the script. If the client is female, then the tour guide should be female. The hypnotherapist can return to the script in future sessions and use some of the ideas introduced in the first session. The script is written below as it would be used in a first session and I have indicated in the guidance notes how some of the sites can be returned to and for what purpose they can be used (e.g. blockages; uncertainty, lack of direction; things that need to be thrown away/finished with; impatience; frustration; anger). It is up to the hypnotherapist if they want to invite the client to get off the bus to explore further during the first session.

The script

I want you to imagine you are standing at a bus stop. You are waiting for the bus to arrive. It is not an ordinary bus – it is a tour bus. A bus that is going to take you on a journey so that you can see things more clearly regarding the loss you have experienced. There are several things you need to know about the tour bus. It only goes forwards – it cannot reverse – it is always travelling forwards. You can only buy a single ticket – there are no return tickets. I want to assure you the tour is very educational. You are going to learn a lot on the tour. Breathe in and out slowly while you wait patiently for the bus. Look down at the pavement – look at the patterns on the pavement. I wonder how many lines you can see. Start counting the

DOI: 10.4324/9781032245706-9

lines on the pavement. As you count the lines you are feeling more and more relaxed. Continuing to breathe slowly in – and then slowly breathing out. That's right.

The tour bus comes into sight. It is a double decker tour bus with an open top upstairs. It is travelling slowly and steadily towards you. Can you see it? It is getting closer now – slowing down – it reaches the bus stop and comes to a halt. The doors open and you step onto the tour bus – you greet the driver and then make your way upstairs to the top of the tour bus. Find yourself a seat so you can get a really good view from the tour bus – you want to see everything very clearly. Make yourself comfortable in your seat. Now the tour bus starts up again and it starts to move slowly forward.

You see the tour guide appear at the top of the stairs. He multi-tasks as he sells tickets for the tour bus as well as being the tour guide. He is extremely knowledgeable about the sights you will see on the tour. He starts taking fares and giving other passengers their tickets. He soon reaches you – buy your ticket now. Remember you can only purchase a single ticket – there are no returns. The tour guide gives you your ticket and also a map of the planned tour, which shows the route the tour bus should travel along.

It is a pleasantly warm day – a good time to take a journey on the tour bus. Look up at the sky – see how blue it is today. Feel the warmth of the sun coming down on your face. The bus is going to take you on a journey you need to experience. Sometimes the tour bus will travel very quickly – at other times it might slow down so you can take a closer look at the sights. You can get on and off the bus at any time – to explore and have a closer look at things. The bus will take you to places you need to visit. The tour guide will point out the things you need to see – he will also tell you things you need to hear. You will see and hear things very clearly – and you may see some things differently. You may very well start to think and feel differently about the things you see and hear. Taking the tour bus will show you the correct route for you – which direction you need to take to go forwards. There is no going backwards. You can get off and get back on the tour bus whenever you like but you are always moving forwards. Everything you see and learn will be stored in your subconscious mind – your memories are important – they are there for you anytime you need them.

You have started the tour – you are on your journey of grief. The tour bus is travelling along – you are looking all around you – you are not quite sure what to look at first because there is so much to see. I wonder if you are looking forward – to the right – or to the left. You just have to do what feels right for you – and go at the speed that is right for you. If you feel the tour bus is going too fast or too slow for you, you can ask the tour guide to speak with the driver in order to change the speed – slow down or speed up. The tour should take place at your own pace.

You are going to travel along a lot of roads – wide roads – narrow roads. All of them will have something to show you. I wonder what are you seeing now as you look around. Remember you can always get off the tour bus at any point and explore further – look in a shop window – go into a shop – a cafe – a museum – a bank – anywhere you want. Off the main roads you will see some alleyways – you might want to explore these too. See what lies behind the closed doors.

(Guidance note: if a hypnotherapist likes to use regression techniques, then in future sessions the closed doors can be returned to and used to look into the past to resolve current issues)

As you are travelling along now look at the road in front – look at the side roads – look at the alleyways. I wonder what you are seeing – what you want to explore.

The tour bus starts slowing down and then it comes to an abrupt halt. You see you that there are some traffic lights ahead, which are on red. They soon turn to amber and then green – so the tour bus continues the tour. The tour guide speaks out over the loudspeaker. He is telling you about some statues on the right hand side of the tour bus. He says these statues are of important people. You look at the statues – they look familiar somehow.

(Guidance note: the statues represent people who are significant to the client e.g. a person they have lost/is missing from their life; a person/people who they hold responsible for causing a loss – perhaps a job; injury. This is a stop on the tour that can be returned to in future sessions to address relationships/people)

The tour continues. As well as becoming more and more aware of what surrounds you and what is passing you by – you are aware that your feelings are changing as you look at things. Some things you see make you happy – some things make you sad – some things make you angry. It is perfectly fine to feel different things on the tour and your thoughts might change too along the way – how you think about things – and how you may change things in the future.

For now though you are enjoying looking at the roads – alleyways – buildings – parks – open spaces. You hear the tour guide's voice coming over the loudspeaker. You listen to the useful information he is giving you. You might find that the tour guide's voice drifts in and out, which does not matter. You will always hear the important things he is telling you. The tour bus is showing you so many different places. You will know the ones you need to visit. Some areas are busy – others are quiet. You suddenly become aware of a lot of loud noises – you see some road works up ahead. The tour bus stops. The noises get louder. There are lots of people about – workmen – pedestrians are watching what is going on – crowds are forming. You feel there is a lot of confusion – no-one seems to know what they are doing. The traffic is blocked – there is a long queue forming of cars – vans – buses – coaches – lorries. Nobody is moving at all – they are stuck – there seems to be no way forward. The noises get louder and louder – the confusion increases.

(Guidance note: the hypnotherapist can pause here or return in a future session to use this part of the script to work on being stuck or confused)

Suddenly someone appears in the road and starts waving their arms about. They start directing the traffic. The blocked traffic starts to move. The tour guide explains over the loudspeaker that the tour bus is being diverted. It is going to have to take a different route from what was planned. You have to wait a little while longer – you have to be patient – calm and relaxed – just waiting for things to get moving again. Then it happens – the tour bus is continuing its journey but going on a different route. The tour continues.

The road works were an obstacle. That gets you thinking about what other obstacles there could be on the road ahead – on the tour. Some roads get closed because they need to be repaired. On other occasions an accident can happen and the road has to be closed temporarily. Water pipes can burst and flood a road. Bumps in a road can be unexpected and shock you – throw you out of your seat. Bumps in a road can make the journey feel uncomfortable – even make you feel unsafe at times. The surface of a road can become uneven over time and sometimes a hole can appear which needs to be avoided.

The tour bus is now going on its new route. It is travelling smoothly again at a steady speed. I wonder what you are noticing on this unplanned route. There is a roundabout up ahead. The tour bus slows down – stops – waits to get on the roundabout – and then it starts off again. It goes round the roundabout but does not take an exit. It goes round again and still does not take an exit. It goes round another time and still does not take an exit. It goes round again and finally takes an exit. The tour guide comes on the loudspeaker again and explains that the driver was unsure which exit to take on the new route – as he has never been this way before. Now he does know the right direction to get to the sites and attractions that need to be seen on the tour.

(Guidance note: the hypnotherapist can pause here or return in a future session to use this part of the script to work on uncertainty; not knowing which direction to take; when a client keeps going round in circles and not making decisions)

You notice as the tour bus continues its journey that there is lot of litter and rubbish on the roads and pavements in this area. It looks very untidy and needs to be cleaned up. As you travel further along you see some bin men collecting rubbish from bins on the road and bags of rubbish left outside shops and down alleyways.

(Guidance note: the hypnotherapist can pause here or return in a future session to use this part of the script to work on issues/problems/situations which still exist and need to be dealt with i.e. tidied up/thrown away)

As the bus continues you see a person waiting at the pedestrian crossing up ahead. They looked annoyed. They are stamping their feet. You sense they are agitated because they have been stopped in their tracks. They cannot cross the road.

(Guidance note: the hypnotherapist can pause here or return in a future session to use this part when a client is impatient or experiencing frustration, agitation)

The tour continues. The tour bus is travelling smoothly. You find you are being rocked gently side to side. It feels so very comforting. Just rocking side to side – rocking side to side. You now know that a tour bus may have a route to follow but sometimes things happen – obstacles can be put in the way. A diversion is needed – a new route has to be found. You may be feeling rather tired now. It can be tiring taking a journey. It can be tiring having to find a different route from the one you planned. It is good to visit places and learn things but it can also be exhausting at times. Especially if you decide to get on and off the tour bus – and you have to climb up and down the stairs of the tour bus.

Whilst you are on your journey of grief it is very important that you look after yourself – take time out at some point every day to relax – and when you do feel tired or exhausted make sure you rest. It does not matter how long the journey takes. You will reach your destination in the end. You will know how many stops you need to take and the areas you need to explore. For now though you can just keep rocking side to side – rocking side to side. It feels so comforting. You can get off the tour bus whenever you are ready and you can always take another tour, buy another ticket but remember you will always travel forwards. The tour bus is always going forwards.

8 Lost and found

Introduction

This script should be used when some hypnotherapy sessions to deal with loss have already taken place. The main objective of the script is for the client to reflect on what they have lost and found on their journey of grief so far. It is also a good way for the hypnotherapist to review the treatment plan which is in place. It is vital for the hypnotherapist when using the script to commend the client on what s/he has achieved to date. Future sessions will enable the client to complete their journey.

The client can find all sort of things when the script is being used. I have included in the last guidance note some typical things clients do regularly find. I have also presented the list in Appendix 8.1 because I think many items on the list could be objectives, which the client hopes to achieve and maybe states this in the initial assessment. These could be written up in a treatment plan.

The script

You have been travelling about on your journey of grief – exploring new places physically and emotionally – having new experiences – new thoughts and feelings. You have been carrying a lot of things around with you in a suitcase. Imagine that suitcase now. Then I want you to imagine that you have lost your suitcase. You are going to the 'Lost and Found' to see if it has been handed in. Imagine that you are walking in a very busy place. There are a lot of other travellers about too. All of them have some sort of luggage with them – either a suitcase – backpack – rucksack – travel bag – sports bag – duffle bag. Look for a sign to the 'Lost and Found' and follow the directions. You will soon see where it is – there will be a big sign above the doorway – saying 'Lost and Found'.

When you are ready – go through the doorway and look around you. You see a counter in front of you. At the side of the counter there is a notice on the wall which says: 'Please ring the bell for help'. Ring the bell and see what happens. Just wait patiently – you need patience when things are lost and

DOI: 10.4324/9781032245706-10

need to be found. A person will appear behind the counter – just be patient. Here they are – a person is standing behind the counter.

(Guidance note: the hypnotherapist should get as much information as possible regarding who the client is seeing. Some prompts follow below)

Are you seeing a man or a woman?
Can you tell me what the person looks like?
What are they wearing?
Do they have a name badge?
Would like to ask the person their name?

Say 'hello' to the person *(use a name if it is known/has been given)* and explain to him/her that you have lost your suitcase. The person says that they are there to help you and asks you to describe what the suitcase looks like. You think about that – the size – the shape – the colour of the suitcase you have been carrying on your journey of grief. You describe the suitcase to the person behind the counter, who then asks if the suitcase has any distinguishing marks or features. What do you tell the person behind the counter about the suitcase?

(Guidance note: the hypnotherapist should wait for a response and discuss)

The person tells you the 'Lost Room' is in the back and s/he will go to look for your suitcase. S/he moves away from the counter and goes to look in the back. You are left alone with your thoughts. You are thinking about your journey of grief and the travels you have been experiencing. What it has been like for you since you lost *(insert what the client has lost i.e. the reason they are attending for hypnotherapy)*.

(Guidance note: the client should be left to think about this in silence initially. Then the hypnotherapist should elicit a response using the questions which follow to discuss in more detail)

What did you expect?
What was unexpected?

The person comes back to the counter and apologises that your suitcase cannot be found in the 'Lost Room'. S/he says it is a shame but sometimes things happen for a reason and maybe you do not need the suitcase or what was in it anymore. S/he asks you what was in the suitcase and asks you to describe in detail every item that has been lost. Before you answer remember you acknowledge that the suitcase has been with you on your journey of grief. You have been carrying a lot of things around with you on this journey. Explain to the person behind the counter what you have lost – what was in the suitcase.

(Guidance note: this is the opportunity for the client to talk about what they have been experiencing on their journey of grief to date. The

hypnotherapist should work with the client to talk about what they feel they have lost but also what they have successfully dealt with. It is vital to commend the client and to give positive reinforcement at this point)

The person behind the counter apologises again for not being able to find your suitcase, but says there is another room at the back – the 'Found Room' which is full of things that have never been reclaimed. S/he wonders if you would like to take a look and find a new suitcase and some things that you might need and things you want for the rest of your journey. S/he explains that in the 'Found Room' you can find very unusual things – not just objects – but things you need and things you want to help you finish your journey – things you need to do – things you want to feel – how you want to be – anything you need or want at all. You want to look in the 'Found Room' because you could find many useful things – things to help you – to inspire you – to encourage you to continue on your journey of grief.

Walk around the counter and go into the 'Found Room' with the person. Look around the room – it is full of things. First of all you need to find something to replace the suitcase you have lost. Have a rummage in the room and find something to put your needs and wants in. Do that now. What have you found?

(Guidance note: the hypnotherapist should wait for a response and discuss)

Now look around the room some more and find the things you need and the things you want. As you find something useful tell me what it is and what purpose it will serve on your journey of grief.

(Guidance note: the hypnotherapist then works with the client to identify their needs and wants. After the client has talked about the item the hypnotherapist will ask the client to put it in the new suitcase [or whatever they are going to use as the new luggage item]. Below is a list of 'typical things' a client might find but extraordinary or unexpected things can be found too)

- Acceptance
- Peace
- Peace of mind
- Tranquillity
- Normality
- Move/look forward
- Hope
- A future
- Contentment
- Security
- Happiness
- *Courage*
- Confidence
- Motivation

- Determination
- Resilience
- Strength
- Companionship
- New thoughts
- New feelings
- New behaviours
- New relationships
- New things
- New lifestyle
- New job
- Aspirations
- Goals, objectives, targets
- Stopped recurring thoughts; moods/swings; feelings
- Let go of things (e.g. the past; anger; bitterness)
- Left the past behind.

You have a new suitcase/luggage and everything you need now to complete your journey of grief. Thank the person who has been helping you in the 'Lost and Found'. Anytime you lose anything in the future you can always come back here and look in the rooms. For now though, you need to resume your journey of grief.

Appendix 8.1: Possible objectives for a client to work towards (in a treatment plan)

- Acceptance
- Peace
- Peace of mind
- Tranquillity
- Normality
- Move/look forward
- Hope
- A future
- Contentment
- Security
- Happiness
- Courage
- Confidence
- Motivation
- Determination
- Resilience
- Strength
- Companionship
- New thoughts
- New feelings
- New behaviours
- New relationships
- New things
- New lifestyle
- New job
- Aspirations
- Goals, objectives, targets
- Stop recurring thoughts; moods/swings; feelings
- Let go of things (e.g. the past; anger; bitterness)
- Leave the past behind.

9 Visualisations for emotional pain

Introduction

Any loss can bring emotional pain, which can at times feel worse than physical pain. In Chapter 6, visualisations were presented to help with the journey of grief. In this chapter seven visualisations are presented to help specifically with emotional pain. The main objective being to acknowledge and accept that the pain will subside. A short general introduction is given below, which can precede any of the following visualisations. The hypnotherapist may choose to use more than one visualisation as appropriate. Alternatively, an individual visualisation can be used as a stand-alone and inserted during any session.

Script: introduction for visualisations

I know you have been feeling a lot of emotional pain recently – since you lost *(insert loss)*. Emotional pain can manifest in different ways but it will subside eventually. I am going to ask you to imagine certain things now which can help you see that pain will go away. Just relax now and get into the trance state – you can do this so well. Just relax every part of your body by breathing in and out very slowly. As your body relaxes your mind relaxes too. Your subconscious mind is going to show you how pain can ease – how pain can subside – how you can become pain free. But first you need to think about what you have lost – how it has made you feel. Keeping thinking about what has happened to you – what you have been experiencing.

1 Sea and waves

Imagine that you are on a ship – a very big ship – that has several masts and different sails blowing in the wind. You are alone on this ship. You feel very alone. Start walking around the deck of the ship. You are thinking about what you have lost – how it has made you feel. Keeping thinking about what has happened to you – what you have been experiencing.

DOI: 10.4324/9781032245706-11

As you are walking around the deck, you look out to the sea. You see the waves – the big waves. Keep thinking about what has happened to you and how you have been feeling. As you are thinking and walking, you notice that the waves are becoming bigger – the sea is becoming very rough. The ship is starting to sway from side to side. You hear the masts of the ship creaking. Everything is unsteady. You stumble – you lose your balance – you fall over. The sea is getting even rougher now. The waves are so big – rising up so high – the sea is so rough. You feel the wind whipping around the ship, the masts and the sails. You hear one of the sails rip. The ship is swaying and rocking – you start to feel sick. Everything around you is in chaos. The ship is losing its way – it has no direction. You hear another sail rip. The masts are still creaking. You feel sick – you feel scared – you feel confused – you do not know what to do – or which direction to take.

The huge waves look scary. They seem so huge – strong – powerful – and overwhelming. Now look out to sea – look at the waves – count how many waves you can see. Look straight out at the waves – you know that the sea will become calm – it will not stay rough for very much longer. The wind is dropping. Keep looking at the waves – they are not rising so high now – see they are becoming smaller – the sea is becoming less rough. The wind is dropping further. The masts are no longer creaking. As the waves become less strong – less powerful – you start to feel better because you know the sea is becoming calmer – you will be able to stand up – walk around the deck without losing your balance or falling over. You will be able to stand upright – you will know which direction you want to walk around the deck. The ship is not swaying or rocking as much – everything is calming down – very soon the ship will be able to get back on course. The sails can and will be repaired. So everything can carry on – going forward – in the right direction – on a calm sea.

2 Thunder and lightning

It is a very dark night in the middle of winter. Imagine that you are standing in the middle of a field – a clear open space. You have a good view of the black sky above you. You are thinking about what you have lost – how it has made you feel. Keeping thinking about what has happened to you – what you have been experiencing. As you are thinking these thoughts you sense that a storm is coming. You feel like a storm has been brewing inside of you for some time now. A storm can create havoc – cause harm – result in damage. Keep thinking about what has happened to you – and how you have been feeling. You sense the storm is very near. The sky seems to go even darker than it is already. You may hear a rumbling sound in the distance. Listen carefully – what do you hear? Another rumbling sound. You sense that it is getting closer. You feel uneasy – unsettled – not knowing what is going to happen. Another rumble – getting closer and closer – louder and louder. You feel uneasy – unsettled – not knowing what is going to happen. Then suddenly there is a flash of lightning in the black sky. Then you see another sharp flash – so bright it lights up the whole sky. It takes over the sky completely for a second and then it is gone – like a stabbing pain – it came without any warning. Suddenly there is a huge bang – thunder. You are standing in the middle of a thunderstorm. Lightning – flashing on and off – like a stabbing pain – never knowing when or where it will strike next. Thunder – so loud – so frightening – moving around – above you – to the side of you.

You are standing in the middle of a thunderstorm. It will not last forever, but you need to walk away from the open space – find somewhere safe to shelter. Do that now – walk to safety. In a short while the thunderstorm will move on and leave you in peace. Sit down and feel safe. Watch the sky – keeping watching as the lightning strikes again – not knowing where you will see it next. You can cope with lightning and its unpredictability – you just wait. The lightning is not striking so often now – like a stabbing pain it has started to ease off. The worst is over. Listen for the thunder now – it is not so loud. The thunder is moving away – it is getting quieter and quieter – it is rumbling into the distance. Both the lightning and the thunder are moving away – leaving the atmosphere around you calm but also fresh. Fresh and ready for new beginnings. Look up now into the black sky and think about the future. See the future you want in the black sky. The future stands out clearly and brightly in the black sky. Watch the future.

3 A power cut

You see a comfortable lounge where somebody lives. It has the usual furniture you might expect to see in a lounge – sofa – chairs – maybe some cushions. There is a television which is switched on and showing something but there is no sound, because some music is playing from somewhere else in the room. It is night-time and the lights are switched on – the room is bright. Heat is coming from the radiators in the room. This is a place where whoever lives here feels safe and comfortable; their daily life can go just as it needs to do as everything feels familiar. Keep looking at that safe and comfortable lounge.

Suddenly everything goes into darkness – everywhere is pitch black. The lights are out. The television screen is blank. The music has stopped playing. The radiators start to cool down. There has been a power cut. All the lights on the street outside have gone out. All the houses on the street are in darkness. This was totally unexpected. When something is unexpected it can cause shock – maybe panic – uncertainty what to do immediately. In a situation like this it is easy to forget where the things which could help are located – like candles and matches. It can be hard to find the way and search in the darkness – things get in the way – and you can bump into things which knock you off course.

We sometimes take things for granted because they are always there. We do not appreciate how much we rely on them and what a big part of our life they are. The electricity in a room is taken for granted – maybe not really appreciated. Electricity is a powerful thing – it can ignite and fuel so many things which give us pleasure. When it is cut suddenly it can be frightening – it can be chaotic. It is important to remain calm and think about what needs to be done and what will help the situation.

Look into the darkness – and as you do so, you feel calm. Think about where some candles and matches might be found. You will know where they are if you take your time to think about it. When you know where they are located go and find them. Now bring them back into the room. Strike a match – light a candle and place it somewhere in the room – you see the room start to light up. Light another candle and the room lights up even more. Light more candles – as many as you need. The candles are a new source of power and energy. Keep lighting candles until the room is really bright and you can see everything very clearly.

4 Sock in the washing machine

I wonder if you lose a lot of socks – you seem to end up with more odd socks than pairs. I want you to imagine that you are looking at a washing machine which is in a kitchen. You see the door on the front of the washing machine. It is closed right now but you can see through the glass and into the drum. You see one sock lying at the bottom of the drum. It is lying there – very still – motionless. A small child comes into the kitchen and walks up to the washing machine. S/he pushes some buttons and the machine starts. Watch what happens to the sock. See how it starts flying about in the empty drum. It is being thrown all over the place as the drum spins round and round. One minute the sock is lying peacefully on the bottom of the drum – then suddenly it is being tossed and turned all over the place. It is on its own – the other sock in the pair is missing – and no other clothing is there to surround the sock. The sock cannot do anything to stop the machine. The sock has to go through the whole washing cycle. All it can do is toss – turn – spin – go with the cycle as it happens. Sometimes water will flood into the drum and the sock will sink – it becomes saturated with water – then completely drowned in the water. The sock will be tossed and turned again in the water. Eventually the water will be emptied out of the machine and then the machine will spin very fast – the sock will be spun around faster and faster. This will happen several times at irregular intervals in the cycle. The sock will be saturated with water – drowned – tossed – turned – spun around.

Eventually the cycle will stop. The machine will spin very fast for one last time. It will then come to a stop and everything will be still again. The sock will come to rest at the bottom of the drum – very damp – tired but ready to dry out. Watch the sock dry out – watch it become restored – ready to be worn and walk through life.

5 Wash away the irritant

Some emotions can be irritants that need to be got rid of. Just imagine that you are sensing something is itching in your eye. You rub it but nothing falls out from your eye. You still sense that feeling of irritation. You rub your eye again – nothing happens. You go to the bathroom and look in the mirror. You cannot see anything in your eye. You pull up the top of your eyelid – still nothing to see – but the itching continues. You pull down the bottom of your eyelid – still nothing to see – but the itching continues. Go to the sink and turn the cold tap on – see the water rushing down into the washbasin. Cup your hands together and catch the rushing water. Splash the water into both your eyes. Cup your hands again and catch the rushing water. Splash the water into both your eyes. Keep splashing water into your eyes and wash the irritant away. Keep splashing and washing away the irritant. Keep splashing and washing – splashing and washing until the itching stops.

6 Pus in a spot

You are looking at yourself in a mirror. You see a little bump on your face. You touch it and realise it could be the start of a spot appearing. Time passes – the next day you are looking at yourself in the mirror again – a spot has appeared. It is red – sore – full of pus. Over the next few days the spot grows bigger and bigger. Watch how it grows – bigger – redder – it is sore and becomes more painful as the pus grows inside it. You want to squeeze it to get rid of the soreness – the pain – the pus – but you resist. You know that the spot has to grow a bit more yet – and it will become more painful. The pus is there for a reason – it is produced by your body when it is fighting infection. Pus is a fluid mixture of dead tissue, cells and bacteria – but it has a purpose. The spot has to grow and grow – it results in redness – soreness – pain and more pus.

You resist squeezing the spot – instead you watch it grow every day – you face it – you deal with it. You do this by bathing and cleansing it – using soothing ointment to heal it. Keep looking in the mirror – the spot is as big as it will ever get – the redness, soreness and pain are at their peak. Then suddenly the pus bursts through the top layer of the spot. You feel such a sense of relief. All the infection oozes out of the spot. All the pain is taken away. Time passes – the next day the spot is smaller – less red – less sore – less painful. The spot is healing. Watch the spot in the mirror as it grows smaller and smaller over the next few days. Watch the spot getting smaller and smaller – the skin is healing – becoming smooth and healthy. Watch until the spot disappears completely.

7 Demolition work

You are looking at a very large building. It is very high indeed – it has lots of floors. The building is very old and it has become dangerous. Bits of the building have started to drop off and fall down into the streets below. The building needs to be demolished and something new, more serviceable built in its place. Although the building is falling to bits now it was once very sturdy and served many useful purposes – but now it is beyond repair.

A group of workmen are standing outside the building. They seem to be waiting for something. There is a rumbling noise and the men turn around. They see a huge crane being driven towards the building and tied to the crane is a huge, heavy weight, wrecking ball. The crane comes forward and parks up by some bulldozers. The workmen are experienced in the work they do – demolition work. They have tried and tested ways to demolish buildings. It is time to begin this demolition job.

Some of the men go to the bulldozers – get in – start them up. They then take the bulldozers around the building and start to demolish things that surround the outside of the building. Bulldozers can dig deep and remove stuff. It is necessary sometimes to prepare the way – remove stuff – before the big impact work takes place. Watch the bulldozers start to dig up trees, soil and anything else that is not needed any longer. The bulldozers then scrape up and clear the debris that has already fallen from the huge building. Watch the bulldozers finish the preparation work – paving the way for the crane and wrecking ball.

Now the crane and wrecking ball move forward towards the building. The crane stops. The wrecking ball is released. Watch it swing towards the building – smash – it hits the building. There is a dent in the outside of the building. Keep watching the wrecking ball – swinging backwards and forwards – denting the building – part of the building starts to crumble. Carry on watching.

The workmen group together – they are shaking their heads. One of them signals to the man working the crane to stop. The wrecking ball keeps swinging – but it slows down – slower and slower and then it stops – it is still. It seems the wrecking ball was not powerful enough to demolish the building completely. It made a good start but something else needs to be used to finish the demolition. The workmen disappear and then reappear with boxes which they take into the building. Time passes. The men come out of the building and regroup. One of the men has a device in his hand. He nods to the rest of the workmen and they all walk away from the building. Wait now – see what happens. You hear a big bang – an explosion – and all the huge building collapses. It only takes a short time for the building to fall down completely. It is no more – just a pile of rubble and debris on the ground.

Time passes. A new building is constructed to replace the old building. Look at where the old building used to stand. See the new building – purpose built – strong – sturdy – well built. Standing high and proud.

10 It's OK to feel…

Introduction

Whatever loss a person experiences there will be some sort of emotional response – even if it is detachment or numbness. Even if it is a minor loss the person will react to it either by thinking about what has been lost, feeling the loss or they will behave in a certain way. The person might not do all three things together; the reaction to the loss may be spread out over time. Hypnotherapy is about working on thoughts, feelings and behaviours; and understanding how they interact. It is helpful to remember this and it gives a useful structure when working with loss and grief. In my own practice I like to use the term 'the journey of grief', because I think it is important to discuss with the client whilst in the conscious state how everyone's journey will be different. The hypnotherapist can make the client aware of the stages of grief as discussed elsewhere (Chapter 6). A person may not experience the stages in a particular order and they may go backwards and forwards between the stages in regard to experiencing emotions. What is vital is that the hypnotherapist keeps emphasising that whatever emotion(s) the client is experiencing then it is right for them to feel that way; it is part of their own personal journey and they should not feel guilty about feeling the way they do.

Some clients find it difficult to express their feelings in the conscious state, but once in the trance state they can talk in depth about how they are feeling and express themselves articulately and with clarity. In Appendix 10.1 I have included a summary of typical emotions and feelings which are talked about when working with various types of losses and working through the journey of grief. Some clients may only experience a few, whereas others will experience many. It is very easy to focus on negative emotions but sometimes a loss which brings a sense of release or relief may result in positive emotions. The list of emotions and feelings presented in Appendix 10.1 below is not exhaustive and is not in any particular order. I have used words which have been expressed to me on a regular basis when working with clients, who have been dealing with a loss. Some hypnotherapists may want to make the appendix into a handout for clients.

DOI: 10.4324/9781032245706-12

The short script which follows below can be used as an introduction to working on specific emotions/feelings. The hypnotherapist can then use their own techniques for achieving this or s/he may choose to use it in conjunction with another script in the book, which has a particular purpose; for example - melting away a feeling (Chapter 16) or digging up a feeling (Chapter 18).

The script

Close your eyes now and start to shut out the world. Focus on you – you are an important person who is currently grieving and going through a hard time. So, now is the time to take some time out and focus on you and what you are feeling.

People deal with a loss in different ways. It is important that a person should grieve in their own way – a way that helps them. Grief manifests itself in different ways too – it makes people do things they might not normally do – they might say things they might not normally say – they might think things they might not normally think. Sometimes grief can make a person feel guilty because they are behaving differently. I want you to know it is OK to feel whatever you are feeling, but I also want you to know that it can be good to vent how you are feeling. You can do this in the conscious state or when in the trance state – just like you are doing now – when you feel relaxed and you know you are perfectly safe.

I want you to take some very deep breaths in and out – and to help you do that really slowly I am going to count up from *1* to *5* and then down from *5* to *1*. Nice and slowly so you can start relaxing. Ready now:

> Breathe in: *1, 2, 3, 4,* and *5*. Breathe out: *5, 4, 3, 2,* and *1* – and again.
> Breathe in: *1, 2, 3, 4,* and *5*. Breathe out: *5, 4, 3, 2,* and *1* – starting to relax.
> Breathe in: *1, 2, 3, 4,* and *5*. Breathe out: *5, 4, 3, 2,* and *1* – really relaxing now.

Now just let your mind drift – relaxing more and more with each breath you take. Just drift and drift. Now as you are drifting, think about how you have felt over the past few days, weeks *(add months if appropriate)*. Think about the things you have had to do – have had to face – the conversations you have had to have. Think about the different feelings you have had at various times. Now tell me what you have been feeling – tell me about the different feelings you have experienced.

(Guidance note: the hypnotherapist should then work with the client to enable discussion about each separate feeling. If there are a lot of feelings to work through, it may be necessary to do this work over several sessions)

You have told me you feel *(insert feeling)*. I want you to know it is OK to feel *(insert feeling)*. It really is. You will work your way through this. There is no need to think it is wrong to feel this way. Grief presents itself in different ways – you need to be able to express your grief in any way it helps you.

Focus on that feeling – *(insert feeling)*.
Tell me what it is like to feel that way.
Can you describe that feeling?
What happens when you feel that way?
What goes through your mind when you are feeling *(insert feeling)*?
What do you do when you are feeling *(insert feeling)*?
Tell me more about this feeling.
What do you want to do about this feeling?
Do you want/need to stay with this feeling?
Do you want to change this feeling now?
How would you like to feel?
What else would you like to feel?

(Guidance note: sometimes the client is not ready to get rid of a feeling because it is helping them with their grief. A client may think losing the feeling is disloyal e.g. not feeling sad anymore; or it is something else that is familiar to them which is going to be lost. Consequently, the hypnotherapist may need to come back to this feeling in future sessions i.e. until the time is right to get rid of it as it no longer serves a purpose)

You know that your thoughts, feeling and behaviours are interlinked. You can change the way you think – the way you feel – and the way you behave. So if you want to get rid of that feeling start thinking about it differently now. You do not have to feel that way forever. You are not dependent on that feeling. It may have helped you up to this point, but now is the time to think differently.

Tell me what you are thinking now.
What are you feeling now?

Well done. You have acknowledged what you have been feeling – acknowledged the purpose of feeling that way through your journey of grief. Remember your journey of grief is unique and it is OK to feel whatever you are feeling. You know you will be able to work with and through any feeling you experience. There is a reason for experiencing them – you know it's OK to feel whatever you feel.

Appendix 10.1: Emotions and feelings

EMOTIONS AND FEELINGS

- Lost
- Lonely
- Upset
- Sad
- Low/depressed
- Abandoned
- Deserted
- Despondent
- Despair
- Angry
- Bitter
- Guilt
- Blame/self-blame
- Resentful
- Obligated
- Dutiful/duty bound
- Responsible
- Vengeful
- Jealous
- Let down
- Cheated
- Betrayed
- Frustrated
- Failed/a failure
- Disappointed
- Shocked
- Disbelief
- Numb
- Detached
- Mistrustful
- Doubtful
- Hatred
- Useless

- Hopeless
- Helpless
- Worthless
- Shame
- Intimidated
- Degraded/degradation
- Humiliation
- Embarrassed
- Redundant
- Purposeless
- Directionless
- Pessimistic
- Anxious
- Scared
- Fearful
- Panic
- Trapped
- Claustrophobic
- Restricted
- Unconfident
- Weak
- Powerless
- Out of control
- Paranoid
- Obsessive
- Intruded upon/invaded
- Relief/relieved
- Free
- Pleased
- Excited
- Optimistic
- Hopeful
- Determined.

11 Opening tulips

Introduction

After experiencing a loss a person can close down completely – s/he goes deep within themselves. There can be any number of reasons for this. Sometimes the person simply does not want to talk about what has happened because it is too painful or they may feel shame or embarrassment about what has happened. The person may fear how others may react or what they might say (e.g. 'I told you he was no good'). After a death, a person might want to protect other people from their grief and avoids talking about the deceased person. Others just simply find it hard to express how they feel verbally in the conscious state. The main objective of the following script is to help the client open up about what they are going through and experiencing. It can encourage discussion about difficult topics or be used to talk to or confront certain people. The script promotes optimism and looking to grow, flourish and thrive. It can also be used purely for relaxation purposes.

The script

Someone is knocking at the door of your house. When you open the door you cannot see anyone but you look down and see that a long cardboard box has been left on the doorstep. Your name is written on the box. Pick it up and bring it inside. Now open the box. Inside you see lots of tulips – the petals are all closed up tight – all different colours – the box is full of radiance. Look at the tulips – then choose just one tulip – a tulip that you would like to hold in your hand.

Hold the tulip in your hand – directly in front of you. The tulip's petals are closed up very tight. It can feel very safe to be closed up for a while but eventually it is good to relax – open out – and flourish. You have been feeling closed down since losing *(insert whatever the loss has been)*. Like the tulip you have been closed – keeping things in – tight within you – covering the inside of you so it cannot be seen. You have closed down – not talked about what you have been thinking – how you

DOI: 10.4324/9781032245706-13

have been feeling. It is perfectly natural do this, but it can help to relax – open up – open out – show what you are feeling – show what is happening inside of you.

Look at the tulip in front of you. The petals are all closed up tight. Look at the beautiful colours you see in front of you – the petals – the strong stem – the long elegant green leaves. See how strong the stem looks – keeping the tulip upright and steady. Right at the bottom of the stem, you see that there is a bulb and roots – they have not been cut off from the tulip.

Focus now on the petals. The more you look at them, you see them start to relax – as they relax you start to feel more relaxed. The petals relax even more and start to open up – very slowly – watch the petals start to open up. As you watch the petals relax and open up – let yourself relax – open yourself up – feel less tight inside and closed within you. It is good to relax – you do not have to remain closed up – you do not have to protect other people. People should know how you are feeling – it is good to express yourself – vent if you need to do so. Keep watching the petals relaxing and opening up more and more. As you watch them opening up – you feel more relaxed – you are opening up – opening up deep inside you. That is starting to feel so good, isn't it? Think of all the things you need to open up about – and let them out – thoughts – feelings – maybe frustrations – regrets *(insert anything else as appropriate)* – let them all out.

(Guidance note: the hypnotherapist should leave plenty of time for the client to talk. Some clients may be very reticent at first if they have been bottling things up for a long time. They should not be rushed. Others immediately gush as though they have been given permission to speak. Some questions follow below for use if required)

What do you want to talk about?
What do you need to talk about?
Is there anything that is difficult for you to talk about?
Are there things you have been keeping to yourself?
Is there anyone you need to speak with?
Is there anything you need to tell someone in particular?
Is there a reason you find it difficult to talk about *(insert as appropriate)*?
Is there a reason you have not told/spoken with/talked about *(insert as appropriate)*?

The tulip is now so relaxed it has completely opened up – now you can see right inside of it. The inside of the tulip is rich in colour. You can also see the little black stamens right in the centre – standing up straight and strong. Just imagine yourself as one of those stamens – standing up straight and strong – open to the world. Open to talking to people. Open to expressing yourself. Open to facing anything that confronts you. Open to experiencing new things in the future. Open to talking about what you have lost – saying how that makes you feel – what you want to happen now – what you want people to do. Open to expressing yourself honestly and clearly.

It is time to face the future – plant the seeds for new beginnings and growth. So look again at the tulip. Focus your attention on the bottom of the stem where you can see the bulb – and then look at the roots hanging downwards. Break off the bulb and roots – hold them in your hand. Imagine you are standing in a garden – you can see a lawn surrounded by borders filled with rich, healthy soil. You may see some plants, flowers, shrubs or bushes. Find a space in one of the borders and nearby you will see a garden trowel. You are going to plant the bulb and roots from the tulip – deep into the rich soil. Dig deep now and as you do so – feel a sense of optimism growing inside of you. The deeper you dig, the more optimistic you feel. Optimistic that you have a bright future – things to look forward to – things you want to do – to see – to experience. You are open to experiencing new things. You are going to grow and flourish. Plant the bulb and roots deep into the soil. You know the bulb and roots will grow – new tulips will grow and flourish – and then they will thrive. You will do the same. Like the tulip you can relax and open up. Like the bulb and roots you will grow and flourish into the future – and then you will thrive.

12 Feeling alone

Introduction

I have said for decades that I think one of the most prevalent and cruellest diseases in the world is that of loneliness. The feeling of being alone is dreadful. I am sure most of us have had the experience of feeling alone even when being surrounded by people but it has only been for a short time. For many people, they carry that feeling with them every moment of their lives.

One of the most common things I work with in my hypnotherapy practice is the loneliness a child or young person experiences after they have been bullied or they have lost their friends. Bullying has always been present in so many different locations and establishments. I am sure everyone can remember someone who was bullied at their own school. With the advances in technology and social media, cyber bullying can be carried out in so many different ways now. Victims of bullying or harassment via social media can feel very exposed and they may feel they have lost their privacy (and maybe their dignity). Since friendship groups have become very popular, young people can experience being excluded by their peer group, who they formerly considered to be their friends. It is a terrible loss which can have both short and long term effects. The most common short-term effect being isolated and feeling alone. In the long-term it may be very difficult to trust people. Consequently making friends can be hard and a person's social circle may be very limited. Of course, adults can experience the same sort of thing, that is, bullying in the workplace or exclusion from groups or clubs.

People who have to leave their home can feel very alone when they have to live amongst strangers. This could be an asylum seeker or refugee living in a detention centre or hostel. A woman fleeing from domestic abuse with her children may welcome the support she receives in a refuge but still has the feeling of being alone – even though she is surrounded by workers, other women and their children.

As people are living longer, older people can find themselves feeling alone when they have lost all their family and friends. Not everyone has a

DOI: 10.4324/9781032245706-14

big family to start with so there are many older people without any living relatives. It is tragic and very sad when an older person's children have died before them. I have heard older people joke about the fact their social life consists of going to funerals. The main aim of any treatment plan will be to explore the feelings being experienced but ultimately to work on having meaningful and trustworthy relationships in the future. Very often this will involve working on low-esteem, building confidence and becoming more assertive.

The main aim of the script is to encourage the development of courage to experience new things. Loneliness is left behind and a sense of belonging and being part of something is experienced.

The script

I know you are feeling very alone right now, but that feeling will not last forever. I want you to know that you can make changes in your life and that you can meet people who you will be able to trust. It is a terrible thing when people let you down – when you are left to feel all alone. People come in and out of your life for a reason, but sometimes you have got to be pro-active and make things happen for you. You can make things happen for you.

I want you to imagine that you are standing outside a huge circle. I do not know where this circle is and it really does not matter – just see a huge circle and you are on standing on the outside of it. As you stand there you feel very alone. There is nobody else around. It is very quiet. It is very still. You feel very alone. Look at the circle – it looks very inviting. Maybe you are wondering what it would like to step into the circle. Because of what has happened to you in the past you may be wary of entering somewhere new – trying something different. It takes courage to try new things.

Keep looking at the circle. Around it – the perimeter – also look inside it. You sense that you are being invited into the circle. I wonder if you are seeing anything in the circle. I wonder what you are sensing. You have courage deep inside you – it has always been there. When you have knock backs in your life it can feel like you have no courage left – but you have – your courage will always be there. You have the courage to make changes in your life and it can start right now – start some new beginnings. Before you do that – you need to get rid of that feeling of loneliness. I want you to feel that sense of being alone for the very last time. Imagine that you take the feeling of loneliness from within you and place it on one of your hands. I wonder what you are seeing in your hand. On the count of *3* you will step into the circle and just before you do so – you will throw whatever you are holding in your hand far away. Be ready to throw far away whatever you are holding in your hand – throw it now – far, far away. Now step into the circle – *1, 2,* and *3* – in you go now.

Immediately you feel different – you feel a shift in yourself. You feel welcomed. You feel a sense of belonging. You feel part of the circle. Now is the time to walk further into the circle and see what you find in it. The circle is your future. Walk around it and find what you want for the future. Tell me what you find.

What are you seeing?
What do you find?
What do you need to do?
Describe to me how you are feeling now.

(Guidance note: the hypnotherapist may wish to finish with some further ego boosting)

13 Fire and anger

Introduction

Anger is a very common emotion that has to be dealt with when someone has experienced a loss or maybe multiple losses. A person who is usually passive or perhaps very tolerant may not show anger externally but that does not mean s/he will not be feeling it. Anger is part of the journey of grief; it will manifest itself in some way at some point. Anger can be viewed as a negative feeling or response to something, but in fact it can be a very positive thing to help someone vent. This should be encouraged as long as there is no likelihood of harm to others. Anger can come and go whilst on the journey of grief, but there will be a time when it needs to come to an end and the hypnotherapist will work on this with a client. The following two scripts will help with ending the anger part of the journey with the use of fire.

Script 1: Blazing trail of fire

I want you to imagine that somehow you are high up in the sky somewhere. Maybe you are sitting on a cloud or flying about on the back of a huge eagle or maybe you are just sitting on the top of a very high mountain. It is an extremely hot day. I do not know, but wherever you are when you look down you can see a huge forest. The forest is very dense – it has existed for many years – it is densely populated with so many trees. Look down now and see all the different types of trees – and as you look you become aware of all the pathways in between the trees. This is a very beautiful forest where many people come to walk. You can see there are many ways to get into the forest and at some of the points of entry bins have been placed so people can put their rubbish in them to keep the forest tidy. However, some people are not very tidy and they dump their rubbish – leaving things that really should be taken home. One pile of rubbish catches your eye because it is shining in the bright sunlight. It is a very hot day today. The bin is full and so things have been left next to it. As you are looking more closely at the bin and the rubbish next to it you see a

DOI: 10.4324/9781032245706-15

cigarette lighter – a box of matches – and an aerosol can. You become aware of the heat – how it is getting hotter – hotter and hotter. The suddenly you see flames by the bin. The rubbish next to the bin has ignited.

Watch the flames – see how they grow. They flicker like the anger that has been inside of you since you lost *(insert loss)*. The flames flicker and then they grow in strength so they grow taller and bigger. The flames grow upwards and as they do so they grow more powerful. Then the flames begin to spread. Just like your anger has spread into your daily life. Sometimes you have become angry about something that was perhaps quite trivial but you got angry. The flames of anger have been flickering inside of you for some time now.

Turn your attention back to the rubbish by the bin and watch the flames. They have become very big and they have started to spread – moving away from the bin. The flames are moving down the pathway – then the flames spread along smaller pathways. The flames keep spreading so what you are watching is a blazing trail of fire. Just like anger, the blazing trail of fire goes in all directions – spreading outwards – and upwards. Watch how the trees are catching fire and as you see this happening it becomes hard to see the pathways anymore because they are just a blazing trail of fire. It is time to take action before the whole forest is completely destroyed. The blazing trail may be hot, strong and powerful but it can be stopped.

Look at the clear blue sky and the sun which is shining so brightly. You are going to take control and make some changes. Make the sun disappear – do that now. Then bring in some clouds – big grey clouds. Make the blue sky turn dark grey. Bring more clouds into the grey sky which is getting darker and darker. Bring in more clouds so it is getting very dark now. Focus on the clouds and start the rain. See the rain start to trickle from some of the clouds – then more rain comes down from some other clouds. The rain is falling onto the forest – the rain will stop the blazing trail of fire. See the rain start to fall more quickly. The rain is becoming heavier and heavier. All the clouds are raining now. You see heavy – torrential rain falling. Look down at the forest. See what the rain is doing to the blazing trail of fire. The fire is being dampened down. The rain is hampering the spread of fire. The rain is dampening down the flames of the fire. The fire is losing its power – it cannot spread out any more. The rain keeps falling harder and harder – stopping the spread of the fire – putting an end to the flames – the burning – the destruction. Feel the strength of the falling rain overpowering the fire. The blazing trail of fire is being cut off – it is being stopped.

Continue to watch as the rain puts out the fire. Feel any anger that is lingering inside of you lose its strength – lose its power – it is dying out. Your anger has served its purpose – you do not need it anymore. It needs to be extinguished completely. Feel it leaving you. Feel the anger being replaced by calmness. You are calm. You have no need to feel angry anymore.

Return your attention to the forest. The blazing trail of fire has been extinguished by the rain completely. You see smoke smouldering upwards from the ground. Parts of the forest have been destroyed – and that is really sad – but the forest can be replanted. New trees can be planted and growth will take place. It will take some time but the forest will grow again. Now that you have let your anger go, you will be able to grow and to flourish. You can plant seeds in your mind to help you start a new way of life. Like the forest you are ready to plant, grow and flourish.

Script 2: The cremation

You have been experiencing bouts of anger for some time now and we under-stand why this is. Anger can help you – it does not have to be a negative thing – it can help you express yourself and get you through things. There comes a time though when you need to go to the next stage of your journey of grief – whatever that will be – you will know. So it is time now to cremate the things that have been making you angry – the things you have been dealing with.

I want you to imagine that you are in a crematorium. You are in a room where the services take place. There is a place at the front where people can speak. There are lots of chairs in rows. Then there is a platform on which coffins can be placed, which has curtains on either side that can be moved around when needed. Walk towards the platform and go around the side of it and you will find a door. Go through the door and you will find yourself in a room where the coffins are burnt in the cremators. As you look around this room you see that there is a coffin lying on a long trolley – the lid of the coffin is on the floor. There is nobody else around so you go to take a closer look at the coffin. I wonder what it is like – whether it is made of wood or whether it is a wicker coffin made of natural materials – or maybe it is a big polished casket. Look at the outside of the coffin and then look at the inside of it. The coffin is empty. See how long the coffin is – how wide it is – how deep it is – so you know how much it could hold.

Take a step back and think about all the things that have been making you angry. Also think about the thoughts you have been having and in addition other negative feelings you may have been experiencing. As you are thinking about these things – see them hovering over the empty coffin. One by one I want you to tell me what you are seeing. Then one by one you are going to put these things in the coffin.

(Guidance note: the hypnotherapist works with the client to look at each thing which has caused the anger; this could be the actual loss; person/ people; situations; what has been said/done. The following questions/ prompts can be used if required)

Tell me what you are seeing above the coffin.
Describe it to me.

How did this *(whatever is being seen)* make you angry?

What were you angry about exactly?

How do feel now you are looking at *(whatever is being seen)*?

Do you need to say/do anything in particular?

Are you ready to put *(whatever is being seen)* in the coffin?

Good – put *(whatever is being seen)* in the coffin now because you have dealt with it.

Now imagine the actual anger hovering over the coffin. Focus on the anger and how it looks.

Describe how anger looks to you.

How do feel as you look at anger?

Do you need to say/do anything in particular?

Are you ready to put anger in the coffin?

Good – put anger in the coffin now because you have dealt with it.

Is there anything else *(e.g. other thoughts/feelings)* still hovering above the coffin?

(Guidance note: if any other thought/feeling is being seen above the coffin the hypnotherapist should repeat as follows until all the thoughts/feelings have been put in the coffin. The hypnotherapist should be prepared for the possibility that other things can appear above the coffin at this stage)

Describe how *(thought/feeling)* looks to you.

How do feel as you look at *(thought/feeling)*?

Do you need to say/do anything in particular?

Are you ready to put *(thought/feeling)* in the coffin?

Good – put *(thought/feeling)* in the coffin now because you have dealt with it.

Is there anything else you want to put in the coffin?

It is time now to put the lid on the coffin. Lift up the lid and put it on top of the coffin. Somewhere in the room you will find a screwdriver. When you have found it screw the lid down – screw it very tight.

There are several cremators in the room. Choose which one the coffin should go in and then open the door. The door has a small window in it. Now push the trolley towards the cremator. Then push the coffin into the cremator and close the door. At the side of the door there is a button which will ignite the cremator. When you are ready – take a deep breath – and push the button. Look through the window on the door. See the flames start to burn in the cremator. Keep watching through the window in the door – watch the coffin and all the things you have put in it burn. Watch the anger – and all the things that caused the anger – burn. As you are watching everything burn – you feel everything you put in the coffin leaving you. You feel lighter and positive. Continue to watch the coffin and everything you placed in it turn to ashes. Burning – smouldering – not existing anymore. Let everything burn away and turn to ashes.

When the cremation has finished take some time to relax. Enjoy the calmness which surrounds you. Calmness in the room – and the calmness deep within you. Just enjoy being calm.

It is time to leave the crematorium now. As you go out of the door somebody hands you an urn. You know the urn contains the ashes from the cremator. What would you like to do with ashes?

(Guidance note: the hypnotherapist then works with the client to dispose of the ashes, but should not be surprised if the client leaves the ashes at the crematorium)

14 Learning to cry

Introduction

Not everyone finds it easy to show or express their emotions. Some generations have been brought up to hide what they are feeling. In Britain for many years the population was expected to 'keep a stiff upper lip'. More recently venting how one feels is encouraged and it is believed that talking about and showing your feelings can be cathartic. Nevertheless, some people still struggle to express themselves and find it extremely difficult to say or show how they feel.

The subject of this chapter is crying, which to some people appears to be a sign of weakness. There is absolutely nothing wrong with crying. Some people can dissolve into tears very easily, others just cannot cry when they need to do so. When someone is bereaved they may say they want to cry but find it impossible. Usually at some point in the future (even years on) something will trigger an expression of grief which involves crying. When I discuss expressing emotion or crying in particular, a question I regularly put to clients is: 'What's the longest time you have cried for?' This usually gets them thinking. The longest duration I have been told is six hours. This is useful information to share and discuss; especially when a client feels it is a weakness to cry even for a few seconds or a minute.

Two scripts are included for use with clients who want or need to cry but find it difficult or impossible to do so. Each script can effectively trigger crying to the benefit of the client. Script 2 is a short visualisation originally designed for working with a child, but it works equally well for an adult.

Script 1: Dambusters

I want you to imagine that you are sitting down on one side of a massively wide river. It is really very wide indeed. Just look at the river flowing in front of you. Then turn your attention to the other side of the river. You suddenly see a huge dam. Look at the dam. It is made of concrete. You

DOI: 10.4324/9781032245706-16

may also see bits of rock and earth within it – look closely. You are amazed at the vastness of the dam – it is such a huge structure. The concrete is strong – doing a good job of confining and controlling the flow of the river.

It is a really hot, sunny day. Excessively hot – it feels like you might be in a desert. Everything around you feels hot and dry – bone dry. It is as though the atmosphere surrounding you is holding its breath – it cannot breathe – it is as though it is waiting for something happen. Focus your attention on the concrete. Imagine how hot that concrete might feel if you touched it. Hot and very dry – yes very dry – it has not rained in a very long time – there has been a drought – but things can change.

Look at the dam. Look how vast it is – how wide it stretches right across the river. Look from one side to the other. Looking at the concrete – see if you can see any patterns – cracks – marks – bits of earth – rocks. Look back again across the dam – from one side to the other. Be aware of how dry the concrete is.

Then look at the top of the dam – how tall it is. See how it reaches down into the river – look downwards – follow the dam from the very top to the very bottom. Look at the concrete – I wonder if you can see any patterns – cracks – marks – bits of earth – rocks. Now look from the bottom of the dam where it reaches into the river and then look upwards to the very top. Be aware of how dry the concrete is.

Look further up now – above the dam – high into the clear blue sky. See the sun shining so brightly – making everything so hot and dry – very dry. You know that you can make things happen with the power of your subconscious mind. So I want you to bring some clouds into the clear blue sky. The clouds you bring in are grey – very grey – and as they travel into the blue sky they become darker and darker. The sky starts to become darker too as the grey clouds travel across it. Everything is becoming darker – cooler – darker and cooler. Feel the change in the atmosphere. It is becoming cooler but you also sense the atmosphere is becoming moist. You feel something drop on your skin – a raindrop. Look at the dark grey clouds – you see rain start to fall onto the dam – the concrete starts to become damp. As you are looking at the speckles of dampness on the concrete, you feel moistness in both your eyes.

Watch the raindrops start to fall more quickly from the clouds onto the dam. The dampness on the concrete looks more like rivulets of water running down the dam. The rain is getting heavier and heavier – the raindrops are falling faster and faster. As you are watching the rain falling down – and running down the dam – you feel a sense of release. The rain is flowing freely – the drought is over. As you enjoy watching the rain you feel the moistness in your eyes become very damp and then you feel your eyes fill up with water – everything becomes very blurred. You realise you have tears in your eyes. The drought is over – it is time to let the tears flow. The rain is coming down really heavy now – down into the river which is flowing faster and faster. Your tears are flowing faster and faster. Feel the tears streaming down your cheeks – onto your mouth – towards your jawbone and chin – and down onto your neck. Watch the river flow and rise – I wonder if the river is going to burst its banks.

Keep watching the rain falling down the dam making its way down into the river. As you watch you feel tears coming out of your eyes and streaming down your cheeks – onto your mouth – towards your jawbone and chin – and down onto your neck. Let your tears flow and fall – flow and fall. Feel that sense of release – as your tears are gushing now – let everything you have been keeping inside you *(insert any emotions a client may have discussed)* come out. Let it all out now. The drought is over – you can cry freely – whenever you need to – as much as you need to. There is no need to keep things inside you – let everything out – into the open. Cry for as long as you want – cry for as long as you need to do so. I shall be silent for a while, so you can cry for as long you want – cry for as long as you need to do so.

(Guidance note: the hypnotherapist must leave the client to cry before going on to work with the emotions which are being released. The client may need to revisit these emotions in future sessions, because it may be necessary to stay with the emotions for longer i.e. until the time is right to release them. This is all part of the grieving process – emotions have to be worked through on the journey of grief. Once the work is complete i.e. the grieving is done, it is important to get rid of the emotion(s) completely. This can be achieved by using the river to take the emotion away)

Well done you have felt that emotion – acknowledged it – and worked through it. Now it is time to let it go forever. So look at the bottom of the dam. Look at the river flowing freely – travelling far into the distance. Now feel that emotion one more time – then imagine throwing it into the river and watch the river take it away. See it flowing away – away – away into the distance until it is out of sight and gone forever. Now focus on the water – the river continues to flow – calmly. The river continues to flow – just as life continues. You feel calm and relaxed – ready to move forward – calm and relaxed.

Script 2: The crying doll

You are holding a doll in your hands. Look at the doll. It looks very like you and funnily enough it is called *(name of client)*. Look at the doll – how sad s/he looks. Look at his/her face. Look at his/her two eyes. Focus on the eyes. You start to see the eyes become misty – glazing over. The eyes start filling up – becoming full of water – you realise *(name of client)* is crying. A few tears trickle down *(name of client)*'s face. More tears come out of *(name of client)*'s eyes. The tears start to stream, so *(name of client)*'s cheeks are saturated by tears.

It is good to cry. There is no shame in showing how you feel. When you have lost someone or something it is only natural to feel sad – upset – and it is good to cry. To vent how you feel. Let it all out. Cry whenever you need to do so.

So watch the *(name of client)* doll – watch him/her cry. Feel the sadness inside of *(name of client)*. Feel the sadness coming out of *(name of client)* – flowing away – ebbing away. Watch those tears fall – streaming down. The sadness is being washed away. Keep watching the *(name of client)* doll – watch until the tears slow down – watch until the tears stop. Watch and wait for the *(name of client)* doll to smile.

15 Wobbling

Introduction

People can feel very panic-stricken when they have lost a person and they cannot remember what that person looks like or what their voice sounded like. They can also feel very guilty. I am talking about people who have been bereaved but also people can have this experience if they have lost someone in a different way. For example, a parent may have left the client when s/he was a child and the client desperately wants to remember something about the parent or bring forward some memories. It can be the other way round too – the person who walked out wants to remember the person they left. It can be so important for a client to remember the good times. This is especially common when someone has gone missing. The person left behind blames him/herself and focuses on the bad experiences and memories. Like a bereaved person the client may experience times when they cannot visualise the missing person or hear their voice, the way they laugh or cry.

The script helps the client to relax and embeds the concept of letting things happen naturally i.e. not forcing things. It also suggests through visualising a jelly that having a wobble and wobbling is a positive thing to do. Once the client is deeply relaxed the hypnotherapist can help the client remember the person they have lost.

The script

I know you have been upset that you cannot remember things about *(name of person who has been lost)* – what s/he looked like – the sound of their voice – things you did together. Sometimes the more you try to remember something – whether it is a person or something that has happened in the past – the more difficult it becomes. This is because you are putting yourself under pressure. You are trying to force things to happen – you are trying too hard. What I want you to think about is that you need to let things happen naturally. You need to relax in order to let things happen naturally. Your subconscious mind will bring things forward when

DOI: 10.4324/9781032245706-17

the time is right to do so. You just need to relax and not to worry – just let things happen naturally.

So let's get you relaxed now – deeply relaxed. Then over the next few days and weeks you can practise self-hypnosis more and more. You will become so good at letting things happen naturally – not forcing anything at all. For now, just concentrate on your breathing. Taking slow, steady breaths in – and then breathe out very slowly. Just do that a few more times. Breathe in – slowly and steadily – and then breathe out very slowly. Keep breathing – slowly and steadily. That's right. You are relaxing more and more with each breath that you take.

Now I do not know if you like to eat jelly – maybe jelly and custard or jelly and ice cream. Actually it does not really matter whether you like to eat jelly or not, but I would like to imagine a jelly. Jellies can be made in moulds so they can come out in all different shapes. I want you to imagine a jelly that has been emptied out of a mould and put on a plate. Look at the jelly. Look at the shape of the jelly. I wonder what colour the jelly is. I wonder if you can see through the jelly. Keep looking at the jelly sitting very still on the plate. Very, very still.

Now I want you to make the jelly wobble. Really, really wobble. It looks like the jelly is becoming all floppy as it wobbles on the plate. As you watch the jelly wobble, just let each part of your own body go all floppy. The jelly has not got a care in the world – it is wobbling and feeling floppy – just like you. You are becoming all floppy – not a care in the world.

You see it is can be good to have a wobble because you can become floppy and relaxed. Sometimes when you have a wobble you might shake, tremble, quiver – maybe even feel like you are vibrating. A wobble will always come to an end and stillness will be restored. Having a wobble can be good – you feel floppy and calm when the wobble has finished. You can really relax and then let things happen naturally.

So look at the jelly again – it is standing very still on the plate. Now make the jelly wobble. It starts to wobble slowly – now it wobbles faster – the jelly is going floppy as it continues to wobble. The jelly keeps wobbling. Now slow the wobbling down – the wobbling is getting slower and slower. The wobbling is really slow now – almost stopping – and now it has stopped. The jelly is very still – very, very still – floppy and calm.

Now that you are feeling very relaxed, I want you to look at the jelly again – very still on the plate. The jelly looks soft but at the same it is actually very sturdy – even after a good wobble. In a moment you are going to walk into the jelly. You will feel very safe as you walk into the jelly – surrounded by the softness of the jelly – relaxing you more and more – making you feel safe. Do that now – start walking towards the jelly – and then walk into the jelly. Go into the jelly now – feeling safe – and go further into the jelly – feeling very safe. When you feel relaxed and safe you can let things happen naturally.

Now you are in the jelly I want you to look around and find somewhere you can sit down. You are just going to let things happen naturally – you will not be forcing anything at all – whatever needs to happen will happen. Things will happen naturally – when the time is right.

Now that you are sitting comfortably, I want you to ask your sub-conscious mind to think about *(name of person who has been lost)*. Just let your mind drift naturally – your subconscious mind will bring forward whatever needs to be brought forward – just letting things happen naturally.

Sometimes things throw us off track and we need to have a wobble. We do not feel like we normally do. We react in a different way. That does not have to be a bad thing. Sometimes we all need to have a wobble. A wobble will always come to an end – when stillness is restored. A wobble coming to an end happens naturally when the time is right. When stillness sur-rounds you – you can let things happen naturally. You do not have to force anything at all.

And that is what will happen regarding *(name of person who has been lost)*. You will remember what s/he looks like. You will remember the sound of his/her voice. You will remember things you did together. All these memories are stored deep in your subconscious mind. They will never be lost. Your subconscious mind does what it thinks is right for you and sometimes it may think it is not the right time for you to remember. But you will remember when you let things happen naturally – do not force things to happen – let things happen naturally.

16 Icicles

Introduction

This script is for any client who feels stuck emotionally. Having experienced some form of loss, the negative emotions and feelings are continuing. So many times a client will say to me 'I just don't feel I can move on' or 'I'll never move' or 'I'm stuck with these feelings'. It is always important to explore the root causes of the feelings and work through them, but ultimately a time will come when a client needs to get rid of the feelings. The main objective of this script is to facilitate the letting go. The way is then opened for the hypnotherapist to help the client plan for the future and to work on their hopes and aspirations. It can be useful to use this script in conjunction with Chapter 31, which is concerned with acceptance and aspirations.

The script

It is the middle of winter and there is snow on the ground. It is freezing cold – icy cold. I want you to imagine that you are standing in front of a house. Although you are wrapped up in a coat, hat, scarf, gloves, socks and boots – you are still feeling cold – icy cold. You may be feeling other things too (*insert other emotions/negative feelings the client has talked about*). You are standing in very deep snow. The snow is surrounding you on all sides. Your boots have sunk deep into the snow. Your feet feel cold – icy and stuck – unable to move. It is as though the snow is dragging you down – and it would be very hard to move your feet and go forward. You feel stuck in the snow.

Look at the house in front of you. Look up – high up – to where you see the gutter. The gutter runs all along the front of the house. You see lots of long, long icicles hanging down from the gutter. Look at one of the icicles – hanging from the gutter – thick and wide at the top – dropping down – down and down – going thinner and thinner until it ends in a very sharp point. If that icicle fell from the gutter that point could cause severe pain and injury to someone or something. A severe

DOI: 10.4324/9781032245706-18

stabbing pain – a physical pain. Physical pain can cause emotional pain – and sometimes emotional pain can result in physical pain. Both kinds of pain can feel overwhelming at times – making a person feel out of control, powerless, lost and uncertain what to do – not knowing how to make the pain go away.

You understand so well the power of your subconscious mind and how you can make things go away if you really want to do so. Sometimes a pain is there for a reason. You have to experience it first in order to heal. You learn from that pain. You become stronger through experiencing the pain. Becoming stronger for the future.

Look at the icicles again – high up – hanging from the gutter. Think about what you have been experiencing and feeling recently (*insert emotions/ negative feelings already discussed with the client in the conscious state*). Look at the hanging icicles again and pick just one icicle to focus on. Think about what you have been feeling. I want you to focus on one feeling. What are you focussing on? Relive that feeling now for the final time. Feel (*insert feeling*) – just one more time – the final time. Really feel it.

Now stay focussed on that icicle. See the icicle start to melt. Look at the top of the icicle – where it is wide, thick and solid. See spots of water appearing on the wide part of the icicle at the very top. Lots of spots of water – more and more of them are appearing. They start to run down the icicle – watch them run down – down and down – to the very sharp point at the bottom of the icicle. As you are watching the spots of water running down you realise that the icicle is melting. Keep watching the top of the icicle melt. Watch the water running down – down and down. The top of the icicle is becoming thinner and thinner. The icicle is becoming weaker and weaker. Just like the feeling of (*insert feeling*) you have been experiencing.

The icicle is becoming weaker and weaker. (*Feeling*) is becoming weaker and weaker. Keep watching the icicle – the water running down to the bottom – to the sharp point. The water drips off the sharp point – dripping away – falling away – out of sight. With each drip that falls, the sharp point becomes weaker and weaker. Less sharp – blunter – dull – less powerful. You are feeling (*insert feeling*) less and less – less and less. (*Feeling*) is losing its power. It is becoming weaker and weaker.

As you continue to watch the icicle melting, you become aware of your feet in the deep snow. They start to feel less cold and icy. They are starting to feel warmer and lighter. You also become aware that your whole body is feeling less cold – less icy. Your body is starting to feel warmer and lighter. Your feet and body are warming up – feeling able to move – not stuck anymore.

Keep watching the icicle. It is getting thinner and thinner – weaker and weaker. It is melting away – it is gradually disappearing. At the same time, your feet are starting to feel lighter and lighter. You are feeling warmer and warmer. The sharp point at the bottom of the icicle is almost invisible now – it is not going to exist for very much longer. At the same time, your feet are feeling even lighter and lighter. You are feeling warmer and warmer.

Keep watching the icicle melting and disappearing. Look at the middle of the icicle – it is hardly visible now – melting away. You feel like you want to move your feet, but not just yet. Keep watching the middle of the icicle – it has almost gone now. Your feet are feeling lighter and lighter – they also feel a bit itchy – eager to move – to move forward. At the same time you keep getting warmer and warmer. Keep watching the icicle as it is getting smaller and smaller – as it melts away. Look at the top of the icicle – where it had been very wide, thick and solid. It has melted and is still melting. It has almost gone completely now. It is no more.

(Guidance note: if more than one feeling is to be dealt with, the client will focus on one icicle and then the process will be repeated using other icicles. All the feelings need to be melted away before the client moves forward in the snow)

Feel the itchiness in your feet – your feet are telling you they are now ready to move. Your feet now feel so light – ready to move – to go forward. You are also still warming up – getting warmer and warmer. On the count of *3*, lift your feet out of the snow. You will lift one foot and go forward – and then lift the other foot and go forward. Ready now – *1, 2*, and *3*. Walk forward – feeling free and warm – feeling whatever you want to feel.

Now you are ready to continue going forward. Free of *(insert feelings)* and anything else that has been holding you back. You are free to do anything you want – go in any direction you want. Enjoy your freedom. The past has happened and you cannot change that, but you can learn from it. Think about the future, experiencing it, enjoying it – being free.

(Guidance note: the hypnotherapist should then embed positive suggestions to help the client to plan for the future; achieve their hopes and aspirations. The hypnotherapist may wish to use Chapter 31 'Acceptance and Aspirations' to do this)

17 Ice skating

Introduction

When you have lost something, you have to learn to live with the loss and the difficulties that come with that. You have to learn to live without whatever you have lost. It is almost like learning a new skill. This is the purpose of introducing the ice skater in this script. By imagining the ice skater on his/her journey round the ice rink, it is suggested that on the journey of grief the client may have some stumbles, slips, trips or falls along the way. Gradually s/he will become more skilled and confident in taking the journey. The objective is to promote the idea of recovery, restoration and balance in life. The ice skater being seen should match the image of the client i.e. boy/girl or man/woman. For the purposes of the script I refer to a woman. The main script presents the ice skater, but the hypnotherapist can go further and take the client on their own journey round the ice rink.

The script

I want you to imagine that you are sitting in an ice skating arena. It is a very big place. People come here to ice skate but ice hockey teams also play here. You are sitting in one of the seats above the ice watching people skating round the rink – both children and adults. Some are skating really fast – others are taking it slowly – some are stumbling a bit – some slip – some trip – and some fall right over onto the ice. You have got a really good view from where you are sitting. You suddenly notice a person *(insert boy/girl or man/woman to match the client)* standing at the side of the rink. She looks very nervous. She moves forward as though to step onto the ice but then takes a step back. She then puts one skate on the ice but then draws it back quickly. She stands very still – just looking forward – focussing on one spot on the ice. It is as though she is frozen too. She stays like that for a while.

The woman then takes a deep breath and steps onto the ice. She slips and grabs hold of the side so she does not fall. She stays standing –

DOI: 10.4324/9781032245706-19

holding the side. She looks so nervous and scared. You notice she is breathing very rapidly. She closes her eyes – you can see she starts to slow down her breathing. She is breathing in and out very slowly – in and out – in and out. She opens her eyes and takes a really deep breath. Then she pushes herself away from the side. She starts to skate. She looks so scared, but she keeps going. Taking small steps – she points her toes outwards and pushes forward – she pushes one foot forward and then pushes the other foot forward – she starts to glide. She looks down at her feet – she bends over slightly. Small steps become bigger steps. The woman is moving forward – she is gliding. She begins to feel less nervous and more confident with every step. Her back becomes straighter – more upright. She is going a little faster now. She lifts her head a little higher instead of looking down at her feet on the ice. She is looking forward. She is feeling less nervous and more confident.

Suddenly, somebody bumps into the woman. She loses her balance and falls heavily onto the ice. She looks shocked and lost. She tries several times to get herself up but she cannot do it. She shuffles on her bottom to the side and then hauls herself up. She looks upset – that person bumping into her was so unexpected. The woman takes some time to calm herself – she is breathing in and out very slowly. Then she takes a deep breath and she goes back out onto the ice. She knows she has to try again. She starts slowly – taking small steps – she points her toes outwards and pushes forward – she pushes one foot forward and then pushes the other foot forward – she starts to glide. Small steps become bigger steps. The woman is moving forward – she is gliding. She begins to feel less nervous and more confident with every step. She is going a little faster now. She lifts her head a little higher instead of looking down at her feet on the ice. She looks forward this time – becoming aware of people around her – ensuring that no-one will bump into her and cause her to fall. She needs to keep her balance. She keeps pointing her toes outward and pushing forward – she pushes one foot forward and then pushes the other foot forward – she is gliding gracefully. She is feeling more and more confident as she skates forward.

Learning to skate is like learning to live with your loss *(insert the client's loss)*. You have to travel along a slippery surface, which can cause you to stumble, slip, trip or fall sometimes. You try to keep your balance – both physically and in your mind – but sometimes the unexpected happens, which causes you to stumble, slip, trip or fall. Sometimes you can catch yourself before you fall all the way down. You learn how to recover from a stumble, slip, trip or fall – it comes from experience. Deep inside you – you know how to restore your balance – you know how to recover. So having a stumble, slip, trip or fall will do you no harm – you will learn how to recover and how to restore your balance.

Turn your attention back to the woman on the ice. See how different she is now – the way she looks – the way she is moving. Her head is held high.

Her back is very straight. Her arms are moving in rhythm as she skates. She is going faster and faster – it is almost as though she is speed skating. Look at her face – she looks so confident – she is smiling and laughing. Now she is spinning around on one spot – faster and faster – there is no stopping her. She is so confident. Then she starts spinning on just one leg. Now she is capable of skating at any speed she wants – slow – fast – and she can go in any direction she wants. She does one final skate round the rink – going more slowly – gliding gracefully – looking confident and knowing exactly what she is doing and where she is going.

(Guidance note: at this point the hypnotherapist can terminate using the script or s/he can take the client on their own journey round the rink using the rest of the script below)

So now it is your turn to have a go at skating round the rink. Make your way down from where you are sitting in the ice skating arena – towards the ice rink. Imagine putting on some ice skates. As you are doing that let your mind think about the journey of grief you are on at the moment regarding the loss of *(insert loss)*. Think about how you have been feeling – sometimes uncertain – unsure – nervous – lacking confidence – not sure what to do next *(if possible insert any emotions the client has discussed)*. Some days you feel a bit better – a bit more positive – and you think you have made progress – learnt from what has happened. Then suddenly you stumble – slip – trip or take a fall – you feel you have skated backwards rather than skating forward. It is OK – you will learn from the stumble, slip, trip or fall. You will recover and restore yourself – you will be balanced. Now are you ready to take to the ice?

Take a deep breath in and then breathe out – now step onto the ice. Push your toes outwards and push one foot forward and then push the other foot forward. That is good – you are skating on the ice. Keep going forward – gliding along. Hold your head up high – keep your back straight – look forward. Great – keep skating – going round and round the rink. As you skate round the rink feel the confidence growing inside of you. Now that you are feeling more confident skating round the rink, think about some of the days when you have not felt so good – you feel you have stumbled, slipped, tripped or fallen. It can be good to learn from these experiences and think about what you did to recover and restore yourself – you will be balanced.

(Guidance note: the hypnotherapist can use the following statements/ questions to work with the client as they continue to ice skate round the rink)

When was the last time you had a bad day?
Have you had a stumble, slip trip or a fall recently/since the last session?
Tell me about the last time you had a *(insert what the client has said)*?
What happened exactly?

How did that make you feel?
How did you behave?
How long did this last?
What did you do during that time?
How did you recover?
What did you do to restore yourself?
What did you learn from that stumble, slip, trip or fall?

I want you to remember that you have so much knowledge and many skills deeply embedded within you. Your subconscious mind knows so much about you and will bring forward your skills when you need them. Remember also you are capable of learning new skills – just like the woman on the ice – she learnt how to skate with confidence. There will always be things around you that might make to stumble, slip, trip or fall but you know you can recover and restore yourself – you will be balanced.

18 Dig it up

Introduction

People keep things to themselves for many different reasons. Sometimes it is because they do not want to bother other people – they feel they could be a burden to someone else. Others may be very private individuals – they just do not want to share anything personal with anybody. They like to keep themselves to themselves. Some people have been brought up in a certain way. They have been told to keep a stiff upper lip and not to show any emotion. There is always a reason why people do not share their thoughts and feelings. Some people deny to themselves how they are feeling because they are frightened of what they might say or do; or they worry about what might happen if they confront a situation, a person or feeling. It can be very easy for a person to bury things so they do not have to face them.

The script's objective is to help a client confront current issues and in addition what they may have buried in their subconscious mind by visiting a cemetery. It is primarily for clients who are:

- Suppressing their feelings
- In denial
- Avoiding confrontation, an issue, person or situation
- Needing to face things which have happened in the past.

If there is more than one issue which needs to be dealt with, it is useful to return to the cemetery over several sessions.

The script

Now I know you have been going through a very difficult time, and that you have been trying to get on with things as best you can. I congratulate you on how you have been doing this, but I think it is time to face certain things now. You are strong enough to do this. You have the courage to do this.

I want you to imagine that you are standing at the gates of a very old cemetery. This is a different type of cemetery from what you might expect.

DOI: 10.4324/9781032245706-20

You might be thinking that the graves contain the bones of people who have died, but in this cemetery the graves contain all sorts of things – things that are buried deep – and maybe have been forgotten. All the graves in the cemetery are very, very old. Everything that has been buried here has been here for a very long time. Some things need to be kept buried because they have found the right place for them to be. However, occasionally some things need to be dug up, looked at properly and placed somewhere new.

When you feel ready, I want you to walk through the gates of the cemetery and start to walk along the pathways. I wonder which way you will go. Go through the gates now. Look in front of you and then look to your right – and then to your left. I wonder what you see. Pathways – lots of headstones – ornaments – grass – flowers – trees. It is very peaceful here in the cemetery but I wonder if you can hear anything. Birds singing from the trees perhaps or maybe they are perched on some of the headstones. Are there any other noises you can hear? Look up at the sky – take some deep breaths in and out – feel ready to explore the cemetery.

You know which way you want to go. You are going to walk towards the grave you need to find. The grave that has things buried deep. Things you need to face. When you are ready start walking. Enjoy the walk – look around you – there are so many things to see. The headstones – so many of them – all different shapes and sizes. Maybe you would like to stop and read what is written on some of them. Just take your time – there is no need to rush. You are feeling calm but at the same time you are feeling that courage deep within you. Courage to face whatever you have to – anything that is buried very deep – but which you know you need to face and confront.

As you walk along I wonder if you see any wildlife. Birds – squirrels – hedgehogs. Keep walking. With every step that you take, you feel the courage rising up inside you. You are feeling stronger and stronger. Ready to face whatever you need to. Keep going. Tell me what you are seeing or sensing around you.

(Guidance note: the hypnotherapist should leave time for the client to describe what they are seeing or sensing around them)

You will know when you have found the grave that you are looking for. Tell me when you have found it. You are standing by the grave. You are looking at the grave. Tell me what it looks like and what surrounds it. I wonder what is written on the headstone. Look closely and read out loud the words written on the headstone. It is time to find what is buried in this grave. Now if you look around you will find a shovel somewhere nearby. Tell me when you have found a shovel to dig with. Now take some deep breaths before you start digging. Breathe in – and then breathe out. And again – breathe in – and then breathe out. Now start digging. Put the shovel into the soil and dig.

As you dig, you feel a sense that you are getting close to something. Keep digging – going deeper and deeper. Going really deep to find what is buried down there. Buried deep – really deep – so well hidden. It has been hidden for a long time. Keep digging – getting closer now – keep digging. Tell me when the shovel hits something. Now reach down and pick up what the shovel has hit.

(Guidance note: all sorts of things can be dug up by the subconscious. It is the job of the hypnotherapist to work with the client to confront the feeling, thought, issue that has been buried and has now been dug up)

What have you dug up?

Hold *(object i.e. whatever has been dug up)* in both your hands and look at it.

How does it make you feel as you look at *(object)*?

Tell *(object)* how it has made you feel recently/in the past.

Tell *(object)* how it is making you feel now.

Do you want to say anything in particular to *(object)*?

How does *(object)* respond?

How are you feeling as you are talking to *(object)*?

Is there anything else you need to say?

Is there anything else you need to do?

As you are talking to *(object)* notice how you are feeling lighter. Notice how you are changing. Feel a shift deep within you.

Now you have dealt with *(object)* – you need to move it. It has served a purpose and now it needs to go somewhere else. You will not have to confront it ever again. What do you want to do with *(object)*? Where should it go so that it does not bother you anymore? OK so do that now – take *(object)* to where it needs to be.

(Guidance note: the hypnotherapist should work with the client to relocate the object. This could be in the cemetery or elsewhere. When the client has finished, the hypnotherapist should proceed to find out if there is anything else that needs to be dealt with in this session or future sessions)

Do you need to keep digging in that grave?

Is there anything else to find down there?

Is there more to confront?

It is important that everything is brought to the surface – to the top of the grave – and then once out of the grave to get a clear view of what has been dug up.

(Guidance note: sometimes more things will be dug up from the same grave but the hypnotherapist should also ask the client whether there is another grave or graves they need to find and dig into. Depending on how the client responds another grave can be visited in the same session or the cemetery can be returned to in future sessions)

Now that you have dealt with everything in that grave, you need to put the soil back into the grave – fill the hole – and close the grave.

Well done you have done a lot of digging today and dug up things you really needed to face. Acknowledge the strength you have deep within you and the courage you have to face difficult people, situations or experiences. Remember and feel that strength and courage and use them for your future benefit whenever you need to do so. For now though, rest a while – relax deeper and deeper. Take a gentle stroll around the cemetery – maybe find a bench and watch what happens in the cemetery – the people – the wildlife. Just rest and relax – deeper and deeper.

19 Trees

Introduction

Research undertaken between 1972 and 1981 by Dr Roger Ulrich proved that patients recovered more quickly from surgery when they had a view out of a window which looked at trees rather than a brick wall[1] and he continued to write about this into the twenty-first century.[2] The image of trees in gardens, parks, woods and forests can serve all sorts of useful purposes in hypnotherapy sessions. The three scripts in this chapter which use trees were written specifically for dealing with loss. The first script aims to deal with feelings. It is so important to stay with feelings and work through them, but there comes a time when the hypnotherapist has to help the client to finish with those feelings. The second script is for a client who feels they have lost their way, purpose and is not grounded anymore. It gives them hope for the future by promoting the idea of re-growth and new roots. The third script focuses the client on any regrets s/he may have and then letting them go.

Script 1: Fell those feelings

It is time to get rid of all those negative feelings you have been experiencing. You have talked about being *(insert whatever feelings have been discussed)*. All feelings, whether positive or negative, have a part to play in life – we learn from them and can benefit from experiencing them. Although sometimes, we might question why we have to experience certain negative feelings – being sad, lonely – or feelings of despair or grief. Negative feelings have to be worked through and understood. However, there comes a time when enough is enough. Certain feelings have served their purpose and it is time for them to go – to be cut off completely. Keeping them – holding onto them – will not help – they will no longer be of any use to you – they serve no purpose – there is no benefit. So I want you to think about the feelings you have been experiencing – the feelings that you no longer need and want to get rid of.

DOI: 10.4324/9781032245706-21

I want you to imagine that you are an expert at felling trees. Trees are beautiful but sometimes parts of them need to be cut back or whole branches need to be cut off completely because they have become unhealthy, diseased or have died. For the tree to continue to grow and flourish some parts needs to be felled. So imagine that you are looking at a tree. It is the middle of winter so its branches are completely bare – no leaves at all to be seen. Think again about the feelings you have been experiencing – the feelings that you no longer need and want to get rid of. Look at the tree again and see each individual feeling carved on a branch of the tree. Tell me what feelings you see carved on the different branches of the tree.

(Guidance note: the hypnotherapist should leave enough time for the client to talk in depth about the feelings)

Now a tree feller has lots of equipment to keep him/herself safe and to do his/her job really well. So get yourself ready. Make sure you have a helmet – headphones because cutting trees can be noisy – gloves – harness – rope – and an electric saw. Good you are ready to go to work. Swing some rope around the trunk of the tree and its branches – then climb up to one of the branches you want to cut down. Look at the feeling carved on the branch. Focus on that branch – look at the feeling carved on the branch. Think about times when you have experienced that feeling. When you are ready, cut that branch down with the electric saw. Cut right through it – it is so quick and easy to do – you do not have any problem at all. Cut through the branch – right through the carving. You are an expert feller – good at the job you do. Making a clean cut. Now watch the branch fall. Good job.

Now go to the next branch you want to cut down. Look at the feeling carved on the branch. Focus on that branch – think about times when you have experienced that feeling. When you are ready, cut that branch down with the electric saw. Cut right through it – it is so quick and easy to do – you do not have any problem at all. Cut through the branch – right through the carving. You are an expert feller – good at the job you do. Making a clean cut. Now watch the branch fall. Good job.

(Guidance note: the hypnotherapist will work through as many feelings as the client has seen carved on the branches)

What an excellent job you have done. You have cut down all those troublesome feelings. Look at the pile of branches on the ground. You need to make them smaller. Now you need to put them into a chipper machine and get those branches chipped. The chipper machine is attached to a lorry. On the front of the machine there is a funnel which feeds into the machine and then out into the back of the lorry. The back of the lorry will catch the chippings as they fly out from the machine. Switch on the chipper machine and start feeding the branches into the funnel on the machine. Hear the loud noises coming from the machine – chipping away at the branches. All those feelings are being chipped away – made smaller and smaller. Watch the chippings come flying out into the back of the lorry. Keep feeding the branches into the funnel and see the chippings come flying out into the back of the lorry. You start to feel different – you feel a shift – all those negative feelings are being chipped away. Wait until all the noises stop – the chipping machine has completed the job. Listen. Wait for the silence (*pause*). Then suddenly you hear the lorry's engine start up. Now watch the lorry drive away – the chippings are going to be taken away forever. As you see the back of the lorry disappear completely, you feel a huge shift deep within you – those feelings have been cut down and disposed of forever.

Now move forward in time – go forward to springtime and look at the tree again. See how it has flourished. The branches and leaves on the tree look healthy and well. They are flourishing having had the branches, which were no longer healthy or of any use, cut off. You are like that tree. You had some feelings that served their purpose for a time, but then they needed to go – they needed to be cut off completely. You can flourish now – now that those branches you do not need anymore have been cut off, chipped and taken away forever. You will continue to flourish through the seasons – just like the tree.

Script 2: The fallen tree

Just keep walking forward and you find yourself in a forest. You are surrounded by very large trees. This is a very old forest – it has been here for hundreds of years. The trees are all different ages – shapes – and sizes. Some have very wide trunks – others have quite thin trunks. Look around you at the trees – the trunks – the branches – and the leaves. It feels very safe here in the forest. The trees are here to protect you. There are many different pathways in between the trees. You can choose whichever way you want to go. Just keep walking. Enjoy the feeling of protection – feeling safe as you walk in between the trees – going deeper into the forest.

As you continue enjoying your walk through the forest, keep looking around you. You are protected and safe. I wonder what you are seeing – what you are hearing – what you are smelling – what you are tasting. You might want to touch the trees – or feel the soft grass beneath your feet. Somewhere in the forest there is a fallen tree – you will come across it in your own time. For now just continue enjoying your walk – feeling protected and safe – enjoying the feeling of protection – enjoying the feeling of safety. There is nothing to be afraid of at all – you feel protected and safe. Keep walking and tell me when you come across the fallen tree.

The tree is lying on the ground. It has fallen and its roots have come right up out of the ground. Look at the roots – totally uprooted – the roots are no longer in the ground. Look at the roots. I wonder how many roots you can see. Look at each individual root. Look at the length of the root – look at its shape. Take your time and look at each individual root. Look at the length of the root – look at its shape. Keep looking at each individual root. All the roots together used to be firmly planted in the ground – holding the tree in place – grounding the tree. No matter how strong a tree is, it can sometimes fall over and be uprooted – like when there are strong gale force winds or lightning strikes or some disease gets embedded in the tree. It can be then the tree falls over – is uprooted – it loses its place in the forest. It is not where it should be – standing high, strong and magnificent; rather it is lying down on the ground uprooted – displaced.

Look at the roots again. Imagine them when they were in the ground – keeping the tree upright and grounded. Imagine how strong those roots were. What a good job they did. Over many years the roots grew deeper and deeper into the ground – going further down and down into the ground. They also spread outwards as the tree grew taller – going far and wide – to keep the tree upright and grounded. Those roots have been there for so many years – keeping the tree upright and grounded. Just like your subconscious mind protects you – keeps you upright – keeps you grounded. Over so many years the tree has seen many things. Just like your subconscious mind will have seen and heard all the things that have happened in your life – and all of those things are stored safely in your subconscious mind. Just like things can happen to a tree in the forest – gale force winds – lightening – disease – and the tree falls over and becomes uprooted – things can happen to you too. Things can happen in life that throw you off your pathway – cause you to lose your footing – make you feel uprooted – things just do not seem the same – you may feel out of place – displaced – you no longer feel strong and upright – you do not feel grounded.

Look at the tree again. Look at the roots again. You see the roots which have been uprooted – look closer and you will see that some roots are still in the ground. The tree will be able to continue to live on through those roots in the ground. Just like you still have roots – you are still grounded – and you can continue on your journey of grief and then the journey through the rest of your life – maybe taking a different pathway. Imagine the roots of the tree growing downwards – spreading outwards – finding new ways underground – becoming stronger as they grow – becoming grounded. Imagine the tree growing upwards. Look at the strong branches – beautiful leaves – the healthy tree. Now it is time for you to spread your roots – find new ways – grow stronger – and become grounded.

Script 3: Leaves falling with regrets

We can all have regrets about things we have said or done – or things we have not said or done. It is important not to spend too much time regretting something when you cannot change the past. So I think it is time to get rid of any regrets you may be harbouring.

I want you to imagine it is autumn. The weather has changed – there is a chill in the air and you can feel the wind blowing. You are walking along a road where there are a lot of trees. Imagine what the leaves on the trees might have looked like during the summer months – all shades of green – shiny and healthy. Now it is autumn the leaves are changing colour. Look around you – you can see different shades of orange, gold and brown. You become aware that the wind is blowing harder now – you feel cold. Some of the leaves are being blown off the trees – they are being carried in the wind. Some of them are falling directly onto the ground.

As you see the leaves flying in the air – dropping to the ground – think about the regrets you have regarding *(insert what the client has been talking about in the conscious state or previous sessions)*. Stop walking now and stand under a tree – choose whichever tree you like. Look up into the branches of the tree and wait for some of the leaves to be blown off the tree. Each leaf that you see being blown in the wind or falling down towards the ground will be carrying one of your regrets. Tell me when you see a leaf start to blow in the wind or fall to the ground. You will know what regret the leaf is carrying Tell me about that regret – let it float in the wind for a while – watch it float and then let it fall to the ground. Now watch for another leaf carrying one of your regrets. Tell me about that regret – let it float in the wind for a while – watch it float and then let it fall to the ground.

(Guidance note: the hypnotherapist works through each regret. For some clients there will only be one or two leaves; for others there may be many more and it may be necessary to deal with these in another session)

There is now a pile of leaves underneath the tree. The pile includes the leaves which have been carrying your regrets. Watch the leaves now – see them change colour – once they were a beautiful shade of green – then as autumn came they turned orange, gold and brown. Watch carefully as they now become dark brown – becoming darker and darker – until they turn black as they rot. It is time to sweep them away completely. So find a brush and a bin bag. Sweep all the leaves into the bin bag. Fill the bag and then knot it tightly. You now need to dispose of the bin bag. What would you like to do with it?

Those regrets will not trouble you anymore. They have served their purpose through the seasons. Now it is time to think about the future seasons. Spring is the season of new beginnings. You can have your spring at any time during the year. What do you want to happen in your spring-time – for your new beginning?

Notes

1 Ulrich, R.S. (1984) 'View through a window may influence recovery from surgery', *Science* Volume 224 Issue 647, 420–421.
2 Ulrich, R.S. (2002) 'Health benefits of gardens in hospitals', paper prepared for *Plants for People* Conference, International Exhibition Floriade 2002. The full paper can be downloaded from: https://www.researchgate.net/publication/252307449_Health_Benefits_of_Gardens_in_Hospitals/link/00b4953a3feb61db65000000/download.

20 Building and breaking down walls

Introduction

The two scripts presented in this chapter have different objectives. Some time ago I wrote a very short script about a wall for pregnant women who might struggle to detach their thoughts from what is being done to them physically when they have an examination or unexpected invasive procedure[1]. The script works really well when imagining building the wall, which then blocks out thinking about the procedure. As with a lot of the scripts I write, they end up with changes, they evolve further and sometimes they develop into completely new scripts. Script 1 evolved from the original short script and its main objective is to stop recurring thoughts when dealing with a loss by building a wall. When a person has experienced a loss it can be very difficult to stop reliving things e.g. events, conversations. Thoughts which keep recurring can become very intrusive and so building a wall will help with this.

Script 2 does the opposite action – the client breaks down a wall. This script is to be used when someone is blocked or is resistant to change; and cannot see any hope for the future.

Script 1: Building a wall

I know you have been having difficulty blocking out those recurring thoughts that keep popping into your mind. You keep dwelling on things and have been finding it hard to cut off. Today we are going to help you to stop those thoughts – push them right away out of your mind and this is how we are going to do it.

I want you to think about the recurring thoughts you have been having. See them in your mind. Then imagine that you are placing these thoughts in front of you. See them in front of you. See them in whatever form you want. However you are seeing those thoughts just push them away with your mind – push them into the distance – push them away from you – do that now. You are now seeing them in the distance.

DOI: 10.4324/9781032245706-22

You now need to build a wall between you and those recurring thoughts. You are going to build a wall that is very strong – very wide – and very high. You are going to build a wall that will never fall down, because it will be so well-built. It will be strong – sturdy – impossible to get through – or penetrate from any direction at all – above – below – or sideways. A wall can be made of different materials – bricks – sand – cement – concrete – stone – all of which help to make the wall strong and impenetrable. So start to gather the materials you need to build a strong – sturdy – impenetrable wall. Find and make a pile of bricks of different shape and sizes. Bags of sand – bags of cement – water – maybe some ready-made concrete blocks. You will also need some machinery – maybe a concrete mixer – tools and equipment to build the wall – so go and find whatever you need to build the strong – sturdy – impenetrable wall.

When you have everything you need lay out the materials – start preparing – get everything ready. Maybe you need to mix some of the materials – the sand – the cement – and water – ready for building the wall. Now find a shovel and start digging into the ground – make a straight line where the wall is going to be built. Dig really deep – remove the ground where the solid foundations are going to be laid – dig down deep. Make the line as long as you need the wall to be. Dig down deep – then dig up the ground – you are preparing to lay the solid foundations – the solid foundations which will keep the wall upright. Keep digging – dig deep into the ground – make the line straight and ready – and tell me when you have finished.

You need to get whatever you have been mixing together into some buckets – ready to pour into the ground. You need to lay the solid foundations. Start filling the ground with concrete now. Then watch it set – see it get harder and harder – the foundations are becoming really solid. The concrete becomes harder and harder. See how hard the concrete becomes – making solid foundations. Bang on the concrete or jump on it – test it out – see how solid it is.

It is time now for you to build the wall. You already know how long the wall is going to be. The wall also needs to be very thick and very high. Think about how you are going to do this and start building your wall. Build from the bottom upwards. Remember you have bricks, cement, concrete and stone. Start building the strong, sturdy and impenetrable wall. You have everything you need – all the resources you need – to build the strong – sturdy – impenetrable wall. As you are building the wall look at those recurring thoughts in the distance. You are blocking them out as you are building the wall. Blocking them out completely. Keep building the wall – go as high as you like – make the wall as thick as you like. Make the wall strong – sturdy – impenetrable – to block out those recurring thoughts. Keep building until you have blocked out everything you do not want see, hear or think about. Tell me when you have finished building the wall.

Now walk backwards – away from the wall. See how high – wide – and thick the wall is. Strong – sturdy – impenetrable. Admire your building skills. You can build anything you want now and in the future. You can block out anything you want to make you feel better – to make you feel safe. Those recurring thoughts are behind the wall forever – far into the distance. If they ever try to penetrate or climb the wall they will not be able to do it. The wall will block them out – stop them. Anytime you want to stop thinking about anything at all just visualise your wall and put the thoughts behind it.

Script 2: Breaking down a wall

I know you have been having a tough time accepting *(insert the loss experienced)*. It may feel at times that you are completely stuck – nothing to look forward to – nothing will change in the future. There may be other times when you wake up and feel like something has changed – like you are about to move on with your life – but then suddenly nothing really seems any different – you are in the same place again. It is important to take time to come to terms with any type of loss – big or small – and work towards accepting the loss. Acceptance is realising that you have lost *(something/someone)* and that you cannot do anything about that, but you can do something about how you feel about the loss – how you think about the loss – and you can do something about how you are going to live your life in the future. At the moment maybe you feel stuck – maybe you feel there are too many obstacles in your way – maybe you are thinking 'What is the point?' Right now we are going to remove whatever is blocking you from accepting that you have lost *(insert the loss)* and that you can move forward. You will live your life in a different way without *(insert the loss)* – you can do that – and you will enjoy life again.

So I want you to imagine that there is a huge wall in front of you. Look at the wall. It is massive – so very high you cannot even see the top of it. So very wide – it seems to stretch for miles to the right of you and miles to the left of you. Keep looking at the wall. It seems like there is no way to climb over it – travel under it – get around it – or move through it. It is right there in front of you – blocking your way. So you need to do something about that. Where there is a problem there is always a solution.

You need to break down this wall – so you can move forward. Think about that for a moment. There could be so many ways to break down this wall. Remember – where there is a problem there is always a solution. I wonder what you could use to destroy this wall – what equipment might you need. You might want to blow it up with dynamite – or maybe knock it down with a bulldozer. There could be so many ways to break down this wall. It is important that you find the right way for you – for you to know how to break down this wall. So take your time – think about how you are going to break down this wall which is stopping you from moving forward. Take your time – no need to rush. When you know – tell me how you are going to break down the wall.

Before you start breaking down the wall, I want you think about how you have been feeling during the last few *(days/weeks/months/years)*. Think about what you have been experiencing – what you have been doing – how you have been feeling – and about what has been stopping you getting on with your life. Just take your time and remember.

(Guidance note: the hypnotherapist should allow sufficient thinking time at this point before continuing with the following question and exploring the answer[s] given)

What has been holding you back?

It is time to break down anything that has been holding you back – preventing you from moving forward. There is nothing to be frightened of – you can do this. You can remove this massive wall by accepting that what has been lost has been lost – it has gone forever – and now is the time to move forward. You can move forward and have a different life. You are ready to do this – take some really deep breaths – prepare yourself. As you keep taking more deep breaths feel the strength inside you – growing and growing – you can do this. You can break down the wall – accept what you have lost *(insert the loss)* and move forward. On the count of *3*, start breaking down the wall – *1, 2,* and *3*.

(Guidance note: the hypnotherapist should ask the client to describe what they are doing as they break down the wall and at the same time embed positivity and encourage the client to look to the future)

You are breaking down the wall. Tell me what is happening. As the wall is coming down tell me what you see or find within the rubble. Tell me more about what was holding you back – look in the rubble.

(Guidance note: once again sufficient time should be left for the client to talk and explain)

As the wall is breaking down further, you are feeling stronger within yourself. You are amazed how strong you are – breaking down this massive wall – the wall that was so high it stopped you seeing anything. Now you can see some of the sky. The wall which went on for miles to the right of you and for miles to the left of you is breaking down. Now you can see directly in front of you – far into the distance – to the right of you and to the left of you. You are feeling stronger and stronger as you break down the wall – feeling strong enough to face the future. The wall is breaking down – the wall is coming down. You start to get a clear view – upwards towards the sky – then directly in front of you and far into the distance – to the right – to the left – all around you. You know what you have lost *(insert the loss)* – you accept *(insert the loss)* has gone forever. By breaking the wall down you now have insight into what has been holding you back – stopping you from moving forward. You are ready to move forward – look to the future.

Keep breaking the wall down until it no longer exists. Tell me when the wall is no more.

Now look at the pile of rubble – the debris – the dust. You need to get rid of it of it all, so there is nothing left to remind you that the wall even existed. How will you get rid of the rubble, debris and dust? OK – get rid of it now. Feel everything being thrown away so there is no evidence that the wall ever existed.

So now you are ready to move on – look to the future. You have a very clear view – look upwards towards the sky – then directly in front of you and far into the distance – to the right – to the left – all around you. Think about the future – what you want to do – where you want to go – your hopes – your goals. There are no limits or boundaries or restrictions to what you can achieve. See in the distance your future – what you want to do – where you want to go – your hopes – your goals. Tell me about everything you are seeing in your new, different life.

(Guidance note: the hypnotherapist then works with the client to set objectives for the future. The hypnotherapist may want to refer to Chapter 31 and use the aspirations questions, list and form presented in Appendix 31.1)

Note

1 See Additional script 2 'The wall' in Chapter 39 'Distraction' in Pritchard, J. (2022) *Hypnotherapy for Pregnancy and Birthing: Scripts for Hypnotherapists.* Abingdon, Oxon: Routledge.

21 Leaving the darkness in the cave

Introduction

Clients who have experienced a loss often talk about 'being in a dark place'. I wrote this script about the cave to help a particular client leave his darkness behind. He had left his country of birth to come to live in the UK at a time when there were still unresolved issues with his parents and his brother, which caused him a great deal of emotional pain and stress. He had not been able to talk to his parents about the fact he felt they favoured his brother. He felt he had lost the opportunity to discuss what had happened regarding his brother; at the same time he felt he had lost his home and country.

Time should be taken to explore what has made a client feel that they are in a dark place, but then to embed the idea that things can change after leaving the darkness behind. The hypnotherapist can choose to work on the past and what has caused the darkness or s/he may prefer to spend more time working on the future. The script can facilitate both ways of working as the main objective is to leave the darkness behind. Some clients can remain in the darkness for quite some time because they do not want to face the fact that things will never be the same again after experiencing the loss. The script embeds the idea that there is always a way out and that change can be good.

The script

I know you have been feeling low and in a very dark place. You have good reason to feel like this – it is totally understandable in the circumstances. It is time now to get rid of this feeling of darkness and feeling trapped in the same place – unable to move forward. You know that you can find a way out. A way out to living your life as you should be living it – the way you want to live it. Yes it may be different, but change can be good.

Just keep breathing nice and slowly as you know how to do so well now. Relax your eyelids – feel them become heavier and heavier – a very pleasant heaviness. Concentrate on looking at the back of your eyelids. This is

DOI: 10.4324/9781032245706-23

something you probably do not do very often – look at the back of our eyelids. As you do so your eyelids will become even heavier. As your eyelids are becoming heavier and heavier, you feel the rest of your face start to relax – and then the rest of your body relaxes too. Everything from the top of your head – down the trunk of your body – down your arms – to your hands and through to the tips of your fingers and thumbs – down through your legs – to your feet and right down to the tips of your toes. Every part of you becomes more and more relaxed.

Now I want you to imagine that you are sitting on a floor in a cave. It is absolutely pitch black. You cannot see a thing. There is absolutely nothing to be scared of at all. Just keep breathing nice and slowly. Keep your breathing steady – so that you feel calm. I know it is very dark in the cave and you cannot see anything, but just keep breathing and focus on the dark. You will start to see different shades of darkness. Darkness is not just black – there are all sorts of different shades of darkness. Just sit comfortably there in the darkness and start to think about everything that has happened since (*insert the loss experienced*) and focus on how you have been feeling. You may have felt like you were in a dark place with the feelings you have had. Experience those feelings in the darkness now. Imagine that all those feelings you have had are surrounding you now. The darkness you have been experiencing is surrounding you now in the cave. Feel the darkness.

I know you have felt in a dark place – just like you are feeling the darkness in this cave right now. Everything is dark – you have felt that there is no way out – as though you are trapped. It can be very scary when you feel trapped and you do not know what to do to make yourself feel better but your subconscious mind knows. Your subconscious mind is always there to help and guide you – to protect you. It might feel like nothing will ever be the same again because you have lost (*insert the loss experienced*). Things will be different – and you can make changes to help you to feel better. You are very resilient – you have survived those feelings in a dark place. You have faced them – you have been dealing with them in your own way. Maybe you feel they have overwhelmed you. Now is the time to get out of the darkness and find a way out of the cave. Before you do that I just want you to think more about how you have been feeling. Focus on the darkness surrounding you. Look deep into the darkness. Tell me what you see.

(Guidance note: it is at this point that the hypnotherapist can choose to get the client out of the darkness or look at the past in depth i.e. what has caused the darkness in relation to the loss experienced. The darkness can be used to encourage the client to talk more about how they have been feeling. The hypnotherapist should be prepared for other things to come out of the darkness i.e. not necessarily related to the particular loss which is currently being worked on)

So now is the time to find your way out of the cave – to get out of the darkness. Take some very deep breaths and look again into the darkness. See the different shades of darkness. Look hard for shapes and patterns within the darkness. You will start to see shapes forming – shapes that will guide you out of the darkness. Take a few more deep breaths. On the count of *3*, I want you stand up – *1*, *2*, and *3*. Up you get now. Feel that strength and determination deep within you to find your way out of this cave.

Instinctively you know which direction you need to go in. Just think about it. Now start walking – in the right direction. You have no fear – you know in which direction you need to go. Remember you are resilient – you can cope with anything you come across on your way out. The cave might feel damp and cold. The ceiling of the cave might feel very low. There may be water and mud on the floor. The floor may be uneven – watch your step. Use the walls to feel your way along. You can deal with any of this. Walk slowly – take one step at a time. There is no need to rush. You can change direction – continue to walk – feel your way out – find your way out. As you walk forward the darkness starts to lighten. The blackness becomes grey. You feel a sense of lightness and brightness within the cave but also within yourself. It is getting lighter and brighter as you keep moving forward.

(Guidance note: this is another point at which the hypnotherapist may choose to take time to work with the client on finding ways of resolving particular issues which have caused the darkness. The hypnotherapist should plan and allow for sufficient time to do this)

Then you see some light – you can see the way out of the cave. Keep going – you are nearly there now. You feel a change in the atmosphere – a change in the air surrounding you. Things feel different. You feel changes within yourself. You feel light – bright – happy and positive *(insert anything else that may be appropriate for the client)*. You are leaving the darkness behind you – far behind you – deep in the cave. Look beyond the entrance of the cave – see the brightness. As you keep going forward tell me what you see exactly.

(Guidance note: as the client leaves the cave the hypnotherapist can choose to undertake more in-depth work on hopes/plans for the future. The session can be concluded with the hypnotherapist embedding positive statements)

22 Deflation, restoration and improvement

Introduction

I personally do not like it when I hear talk about a person being 'broken' or 'needing to be fixed'. I prefer to think about restoring a person to their former strengths and working on improvements, that is, to become even better. There will be some losses experienced in life which result in a person feeling let down and very deflated. This is particularly true when they feel a person they trusted has let them down. Typical examples being:

- A friend not being supportive; doing something unexpected.
- Not getting a job; being passed over for promotion (when a manager had indicated it was a sure thing)
- So many things being experienced at the same time result in losing one's sense of being, purpose, and direction.

The end result can be that the person can lose trust in people, but also in him/herself.

Two scripts are presented to help restoration (e.g. of trust, faith, hope, optimism) and improvement for the future (with a brighter outlook – planning for the future, setting goals/objectives). The first script is for an adult who has been let down. The second one is for a child who may have lost his/her confidence for whatever reason and is especially helpful when a child is struggling at school to learn or with a particular subject.

Script 1: For adults – the lilo

Imagine that you are walking along a beautiful beach. You are just alone with your thoughts – thinking about what has been happening recently. No-one else is there – you have the beach all to yourself. In the distance you see a pile of something lying on the beach. You are not too sure what it is exactly, but you would like to know – so just

DOI: 10.4324/9781032245706-24

keep walking along the beach. As you get closer you see the colour of the pile of whatever it is. Keep walking – you are getting nearer to the pile. Some of the pile is also spread out a little on the sand – part of it is very flat. You are getting closer now – you see it is a lilo that is piled up on the sand – it is totally deflated. All the air which kept it firm and smooth has gone. It no longer has the strength inside to support anyone on the water.

Go and have a closer look – you are intrigued to look at the different shapes you see – how the lilo has become out of shape and distorted. Part of the lilo looks crinkled and scrunched up – other parts are flat – flat as a pancake. Go and have a closer look. You may see some little holes or tears in the lilo from where the air got out. The lilo is completely deflated – it has lost all its air – firmness – smoothness – strength and support. It can no longer support anyone to lie comfortably on it. It can no longer float or move on the water.

Things happen in life which can make you feel a bit like that lilo. You feel deflated – let down – not able to function as you should. Recently you have *(insert loss/experience)* and you have said you have felt *(e.g. let down; flat; old; redundant; useless; worthless or insert any other emotion/feeling the client has mentioned)*. Now is the time to think about the future and how you can restore yourself – inflate yourself with whatever you need – so you can get back to functioning as you should.

Look at the lilo again. Think about how you are going to repair the lilo. Have a look around you – explore the beach – find what you need to repair the holes and tears. You are resourceful – you are able to find things and then use them. Do that now – find what you need to restore the lilo so it can be inflated and do the job it is supposed to do. Look for what you need. Now start repairing the lilo. Repair the holes. Repair the tears. Make the lilo strong again – strong enough to hold and support someone – strong enough to float and move across the water.

Now that the holes and tears have been repaired, step back and look at the lilo. It needs to be filled with air to make the head rest and panels inflate. So that it becomes firm – smooth – strong and supportive. Imagine air being pumped into the lilo. See how it starts to lift up a little bit – watch how the panels and head rest fill up and expand – getting bigger and bigger. Filling up and up – getting bigger – expanding – growing – becoming firmer – smoother – stronger. Getting bigger and bigger – being restored to its former strength and ability. Then suddenly it is full of air – restored to its former self – capable of doing what it needs to do. The lilo is ready to go into the sea – to float and move on the water. The lilo will not sink – it is completely restored.

Imagine again the pile of deflated lilo on the beach. Think about how you have been feeling – let down and deflated – like the lilo. Think about what you need to restore yourself and prepare yourself for the future. Look at the lilo it needs to be restored. You need to be restored. In fact you can be even better than you were before. I wonder what needs to be done.

(Guidance note: the hypnotherapist should then work with the client to put things into the lilo and see it grow. As the following prompts are used whatever the client identifies should be put into the lilo)

Tell me what you need to do in order to:

- Feel better
- Build yourself back up
- Restore yourself
- Build your confidence/self-belief
- Improve yourself
- Prepare yourself for the future.

(Guidance note: the hypnotherapist should keep repeating the following questions/prompts/statements)

What is the next thing you need to put in the lilo?
Tell me more about that.
Put that in the lilo now.
Good – see how the lilo is getting bigger – expanding – growing – becoming firmer – smoother – stronger. Getting bigger and bigger – being restored to its former strength and ability.
Feel *(whatever has been put in the lilo)* growing inside you – getting bigger – expanding – growing – becoming firmer – smoother – stronger.
You are being restored to your former self/strength. You can achieve anything you really want to do.
You can be even better than you were before. You can achieve anything you really want to do.
You can do new exciting things. You can achieve anything you really want to do.

(Guidance note: the hypnotherapist should keep working with the client until everything has been put in the lilo and it is fully inflated)

Well done – you have done a great job in restoring yourself and improving yourself. Now it is time to think about the future – plan for the future – and prepare yourself for the future. Feel that confidence inside you. Feel that excitement when you think about the future – and all the possibilities and opportunities it holds for you. Now go and pick up the lilo – walk to the water's edge. Look out across the water – feel that confidence – excitement – and see all your hopes for the future. Walk into the water – go deeper and deeper – until you are deep enough to put the lilo on the water – then climb onto the lilo. Lie back and float – relax – as you imagine the future – you are feeling confident and excited.

(Guidance note: the hypnotherapist should then help the client to set goals/objectives for the future and keep embedding the idea of being restored and improved)

You can be even better than you were before. You can achieve anything you really want to do. You can do new exciting things. You can achieve anything you really want to do.

Script 2: For children – swimming ring and arm bands

(Guidance note: this script was written for children who can swim, therefore, the hypnotherapist should check out whether the child can swim or not before using this script)

I know you have not been feeling like yourself lately and you do not believe you can do/learn certain things. You feel unsure, uncertain *(and insert any other words the child may have used)* and maybe a bit scared of trying things. When you find something difficult it is important to keep trying and practising. You have got to build yourself up and prepare yourself – and find things to help you. If you really want to do something you will be able to do it – you need to believe you can do it.

Can you remember a time before you knew how to swim? Just let your special mind drift back to the time before you could swim. Maybe you are imagining a swimming pool – a beach – somewhere you might be able to swim. At that time you could not swim and even though you liked the idea of being in the water and able to swim – it was a little bit scary and you did not want to look silly to other people not being able to swim.

Remember now how you did learn to swim. What did you have to help you? Someone gave you things to help you. First of all you were given appropriate clothes to wear – maybe *(insert as appropriate: trunks – or shorts and t-shirt – a swimming costume)*. Then maybe you were given other things to help you and keep you safe – a swimming ring – arm bands or a float. Let your special mind imagine a swimming ring and arm bands now. See them in front of you – tell me what they look like – what colours do you see?

As you are looking at the swimming ring and arm bands I want you to touch them and decide whether they need some air putting in them. You want them to be full of air to give you all the help and support you need. So yes they might need a bit more air putting in them because they have become a bit soft as some of the air has been let out. They have been doing a good job previously so might need a top up of air for them to be strong in the future. Before you put in some more air, I want you to think about what you have been feeling/worrying about *(insert the specific loss or issue)* and what you need help with. Whilst you are thinking about that/

those things, I want you to take a huge deep breath and then blow hard into the swimming ring. That's right – do that again – take a huge deep breath and then blow hard into the swimming ring. See the swimming ring getting bigger as you blow into it – getting bigger and stronger. Keep doing that and as you blow into the swimming ring blow in the things you need *(pause)*. Tell me what you have been blowing into the swimming ring. Does anything else need to be blown in? Well done.

Now look at the arm bands and think about what else you might need to help you. Start blowing into the arm bands. See the arm bands getting bigger and stronger as you blow into each one. Keep doing that and as you blow into each arm band blow in the things you need *(pause)*. Tell me what you have been blowing into the swimming arm bands. Does anything else need to be blown in? Well done.

Anytime in the future when you are feeling a bit unsure – a bit uncertain – worried that you cannot do something *(or insert anything else as appropriate)* – let your special mind imagine the swimming ring and the arm bands. Then imagine that you are putting the swimming ring around your middle – that feels so good – in place to keep you safe. Then put the arm bands on. Put one arm band on first – that feels so good – in place to keep you safe. Now put the other arm band on – that feels so good – in place to keep you safe. With the swimming ring around you and the arm bands on your arms – you are not going to sink or look silly in any way at all. You are prepared – prepared to go for a swim. You are going to swim. Imagine dipping your toes in the water first – feel the temperature of the water. Now ready – feeling strong and confident – in you go – in the water and start to swim. Look at how well you can swim – moving through the water. So once you could not swim – then you learnt how to swim. Now you can learn to do other things too – or be a way you want to be – feel confident and proud of yourself. Just remember to imagine your swimming ring and arm bands any time you need some help.

23 Egg timer

Introduction

The purpose of this script is to give the client a way of making time pass more quickly or more slowly. When on a journey of grief, there will be times when someone just wants things to be over and done with. For example, when a person has died, somebody might be dreading the funeral and wants to get it out of the way as soon as possible. It can be very hard when a funeral has to be delayed either because a body cannot be released (e.g. a post-mortem needs to take place; there is police investigation into the death) or in winter there are long delays because of the increase in deaths. This situation has become more common with the Covid-19 pandemic when even more delays have been caused. An added problem being with the restrictions on attendance at funerals during the lockdown, some people have not been able to say their 'good-byes' as they would have liked to do.

At other times, there is a need to slow things down. It can be important to a client to savour a particular memory (or many memories) of a person or of a situation (e.g. a job that brought satisfaction). A client can fear they are going to forget a person or the good times experienced. A client who is terminally ill may feel that time is running out for them and they want to slow things down. This script can empower a client to feel that they can still be in control by slowing things down during the course of a normal day.

The script

You and your subconscious mind are able to make time pass more quickly or more slowly – just as you wish. There will be times in your life when you want to savour a moment or an experience – make it last forever. There will be other times when you just want to get something over and done with very quickly. The journey of grief moves at a different pace for each individual person – it will take as long as it needs to do so. There is no right time or wrong time to feel or do things. You need to move

DOI: 10.4324/9781032245706-25

through your own journey grief – at your pace. There may be times when you do want time to go more quickly in order to move on from feeling a certain way – there are ways you can do this.

Just make yourself comfortable. Let your mind relax – let your thoughts relax – let all the inside of you relax – and let all around the outside of you relax. As you are becoming more and more relaxed imagine that you are looking at an old fashioned egg timer standing on a table in front of you. The egg timer has two glass bulbs – they look likes cones – oval shaped. One glass bulb is on top of the glass bulb underneath. In between the two glass bulbs there is a narrow neck. Look at the glass bulb underneath the narrow neck – look into the very bottom of it and you will see some sand. The sand can measure time. Pick up the egg timer and look at it more closely. Hold it very still in your hand. Look at the sand lying very still in the bottom glass bulb – lying still. As you look deep into the sand you feel still and calm. The sand is made of tiny grains – there could be up to 250,000 grains of sand in that glass bulb – you could start counting them if you wanted to do so.

The sand measures time. Time can move quickly or slowly. Turn the egg timer upside down – so the bottom glass bulb is now the top glass bulb. Put the egg timer back on the table. Watch the sand start to move downwards towards the narrow neck of the egg timer – watch the sand – the tiny grains of sand – move from the top glass bulb down towards the narrow neck – through the narrow neck – and down into the bottom glass bulb. Keep watching the tiny grains of sand moving – down and down and down– through the narrow neck – down and down and down – into the bottom glass bulb. Keep watching the movement, until every single tiny grain of sand has gone through the narrow neck, and all the sand is lying still at the bottom of the glass bulb. Still and calm.

Making time pass quickly

Just imagine now that you want to make time pass more quickly. Turn the egg timer upside down again and start to watch the sand moving downwards – towards the narrow neck of the egg timer – just as you did before. Make the sand move quicker – quicker and quicker. Every single tiny grain is travelling really quickly towards the narrow neck and then passes really quickly – through the neck – and into the bottom glass bulb. Make the sand travel even quicker now – quicker and quicker – it is racing through the glass bulbs. Time is passing so quickly – time is going faster and faster – racing through the glass bulbs. Wow – all the sand has passed through the egg timer so quickly.

See if you can make it go even faster now – turn the egg timer upside down again. Watch the sand moving downwards – towards the narrow neck. Make the sand move even quicker now – quicker and quicker. Every single tiny grain is travelling really quickly towards the narrow neck and then passes really quickly – through the neck – and into the bottom glass bulb. Make the sand travel even quicker now – quicker and quicker – it is rushing through the egg timer. Time is passing so quickly – time is going faster and faster – racing faster and faster.

You know it is important to acknowledge how you are feeling and that sometimes you have to work through a feeling in order to release it. There are times when you just want time to pass quickly so you can feel something else – you want to move on through the stages of grieving. Anytime you are feeling a certain way *(or insert a particular emotion the client has been feeling)* – and you want to move on from that feeling – use the egg timer to make time pass more quickly. Visualise the feeling – see it actually sitting in the egg timer. Then feel it racing away from you as you watch the sand travelling through the egg timer. It is leaving you very quickly as the sand travels through the egg timer. When the sand stops – the feeling has gone – left you completely.

Making time pass slowly

Just imagine now that you want time to make time pass more slowly. Turn the egg timer upside down again and start to watch the sand moving downwards – towards the narrow neck of the egg timer – just as you did before. Make the sand move slowly – very slowly. Slow the sand down – watch the sand moving in slow motion. Every single grain is travelling really slowly towards the narrow neck – through the neck – and then passes even more slowly into the bottom glass bulb. Make the sand travel even more slowly now – slower and slower – it is moving in slow motion through the glass bulbs. Time is passing so slowly – time is going slower and slower. The sand takes its time to pass through the egg timer ever so slowly. See if you can make it go even slower now – turn the egg timer upside down again. Watch the sand moving downwards – towards the narrow neck. Make the sand move even slower now – slower and slower. Every single grain is travelling really slowly towards the narrow neck – through the neck – and then passes really slowly into the bottom glass bulb. Make the sand travel even slower now – slower and slower – watch the sand in slow motion. Time is passing so slowly – time is passing slower and slower.

Sometimes a good memory comes into your mind. You may remember a person – an experience or particular event – something that was said or done. The memory makes you feel good – happy – it may comfort you. You may want to relive the memory over and over and as you do that you might choose to slow down each moment of that memory – savour every moment – and to do that you can use your egg timer. Use your egg timer to slow time down and enjoy the memory.

Part III
Facing and dealing with death

24 Planning for death

Introduction

In my hypnotherapy practice I work with people from all different age groups. Consequently, it would be not unusual for me to be working with a client who is pregnant and I am teaching hypnobirthing; and in the same week or month I could be working with an older person who is terminally ill. A pregnant woman (and her birthing partner if she has one) will be encouraged to plan ahead for the birth of her baby and she will usually have a birthing plan in place, which is written down. Generally, people would tell a pregnant woman that she had done a good thing – planning for the birth of her baby. So why should planning for death be any different? Yet people can be horrified when you mention planning for death and having a plan written in some format – on paper or electronically. People may feel more comfortable talking about living wills and advance directives because they are usually written years in advance of a death.

When people feel uncomfortable talking about death and dying it can make it difficult for a terminally ill child or adult to bring up the subject of what they want to happen – leading up to the death and afterwards. It is often easier for the terminally ill person to talk to a professional or even a complete stranger than it is to talk to a family member or friend. A hypnotherapist could be just the right person to help a terminally ill person plan for their death. This can be done in the conscious state or in the trance state – or a combination of both. When a terminally ill person finds it difficult to talk about their death, I think it is better to do most of the work in the trance state after an initial chat about how the session will be undertaken. Explanation needs to be given about:

- Objective: to think about facing death and dying whilst in trance
- Identifying the needs and wants of the terminally ill person
- How the hypnotherapist will work i.e. asking some questions/prompts
- The hypnotherapist will be taking notes, which can be written up as a plan for death after the session.

DOI: 10.4324/9781032245706-27

What follows is a script which will get the terminally ill person into trance and introduce the idea of developing a plan; this is followed by a series of questions which the hypnotherapist can use to prompt the terminally ill person. The hypnotherapist may feel some questions are not relevant to their client. The same questions are presented in Appendix 24.1, which can be used to write up the plan after the trance work has been done or if the work is going to be done in the conscious state.

The script is written for a person who is terminally ill, but it can be adapted for a healthy person, who just wants to plan ahead. I recently did this for a couple – both of whom are fit and healthy, but the wife was concerned that she needed to know what to do about her husband's business matters in the event of his sudden death. This had been playing on her mind – who to contact, how current stock and goods being stored for customers should be disposed of and what to do with records and registers. She found it difficult to get her husband to talk about this but he did agree to participate in a meeting where the wife's concerns were dealt with. In the same session they both discussed what they wanted to happen at the point of death and for their respective funerals. Another typical scenario for someone who is not currently ill is planning ahead so specific their wishes are made known to family members who may live a long way away and will have the responsibility for organising a funeral when the time comes. Appendix 24.1 can be used for this purpose, but not all sections/questions will be relevant.

The script

Close your eyes and start breathing very slowly and very deeply. Slowly and deeply – that's right. Just relax. You know that going into trance can relax you – distract you – take you to wonderful places. Today I want you to get into a really deep relaxed state – deeper than you have ever been before. Let any sounds you may hear inside the room or outside the room just drift away so they do not bother you at all. Going deeper and deeper now – more and more relaxed – that feels so good.

Now it can be a difficult thing to talk about death but you know and have accepted that you are terminally ill – you are facing death – and you are facing this with such courage. Whilst you are experiencing this wonderful sense of being completely relaxed, it would be good to let your subconscious mind consider what you want to happen as you are facing and preparing for death – immediately after you have died – and where and how you would like to finally rest. So keep breathing slowly – going deeper and deeper again – feeling so relaxed.

It is only natural that you may have some fears about dying – but I want you to acknowledge that you have so much strength deep within you – you are so strong that you can do anything you want. You can deal with anything you have to face with confidence because of the strength that is deep within you. Very like a knight in shining armour – ready for battle – sitting proudly on a horse – ready to face anything that comes at him. Visualise that knight now. You can use self-hypnosis to help with any pain – physical or emotional – you have the strength and determination to look at death and face it directly.

As you are going deeper and deeper still, think about what you want to happen and also what you do not want to happen.

Leading up to/preparing for death

- Is there anything you want to happen regarding:

  - Your treatment
  - Your care
  - Who you talk to/get advice/support from
  - Anything you need/want
  - Anything you need to sort out
  - Anything that must **not** be done

- Is there anything else you need to do before you die? *(e.g. speak to anyone; write a letter(s); record/film a message)*

The actual time of dying/death

- Where would you prefer to die? (*e.g. home, hospital or hospice*)
- Is there anyone in particular you want to be with you?
- Is there anyone who should **not** be in the room?
- Does any ritual or ceremony need to be performed?
- Do you want anything in particular to be done whilst you are in the final stages of dying? (*e.g. someone to read to you; music playing in the background*)
- Is there anything that should **not** be done?
- Are there any words or phrases that might annoy you or irritate you?
- When might you want to be silent/others to be silent?

After death

- Should anything be done immediately after you have died (*this is so important if someone follows a particular religion or has specific beliefs. For example, it may be necessary to open a window immediately after death so the soul can leave or it may be required that only a family member can touch the body*)
- Should anyone in particular be informed about your death (*this can be very important when there are any family conflicts e.g. two sets of children because of divorce and remarriages*)

- What do you want to happen to your physical remains? (*some people may want to donate organs to help other people or to donate their body for medical research*)
- Do you want to be buried or cremated?
- Do you have any specific requests regarding:

  - Type of coffin
  - Clothing: how you want to be dressed
  - Jewellery: to be worn
  - Anything to be placed in the coffin

- Do you want a funeral service or some other type of ceremony? If yes:

  - Where should this take place? (*e.g. church, crematorium, elsewhere*)
  - Who should conduct the service/ceremony?
  - Who should be invited to attend?
  - Should anyone not attend?
  - What do you want to happen during the service/ceremony? (*e.g. hymns/ songs/tunes; speakers/musicians/actors; readings/poetry/anecdotes*)
  - Do you want flowers?
  - Do you want donations to be made? (*e.g. to specific organisations, charities*)
  - Place for burial (*e.g. cemetery; woodland burial; specific plot*)
  - Location for cremation.
  - Are there any particular words, pictures, symbols that should be on a headstone/plaque?
  - If cremated, what should be done with the ashes?

- Should there be a wake/party after the service?
- Is there anything else you need to do in preparation for your eventual death?

Well done. You have given a lot of thought to facing death today. Just relax some more now – you deserve some true rest. As the subconscious mind relaxes more it often works even better. So as you relax more and more your subconscious mind might think of more things you need as you are facing death – more do's and don'ts for your plan. Remember to keep feeling that strength deep inside you and visualise that knight in shining armour – ready for battle – sitting proudly on a horse – ready to face anything that comes at him. For now though, just relax – take some time before coming back to the conscious state. Just relax – until you hear me say your name.

Appendix 24.1: Questionnaire for developing a death plan

Strictly Confidential

QUESTIONNAIRE: DEATH PLAN

Name of client: Date of Birth:
Address:
Telephone/mobile:
E-mail address:

Leading up to/preparing for death

- Is there anything you want to happen regarding:

  - Your treatment
  - Your care
  - Who you talk to/get advice/support from
  - Anything you need/want
  - Anything you need to sort out
  - Anything that must **not** be done

- Is there anything else you need to do before you die? (*e.g. speak to anyone; write a letter(s); record/film a message*)

The actual time of dying/death

- Where would you prefer to die? (*e.g. home, hospital or hospice*)
- Is there anyone in particular you want to be with you?
- Is there anyone who should **not** be in the room?
- Does any ritual or ceremony need to be performed?
- Do you want anything in particular to be done whilst you are in the final stages of dying? (*e.g. someone to read to you; music playing in the background*)
- Is there anything that should **not** be done?
- Are there any words or phrases that might annoy you or irritate you?
- When might you want to be silent/others to be silent?

After death

- Should anything be done immediately after you have died (*this is so important if someone follows a particular religion or has specific beliefs. For example, it may be necessary to open a window immediately after death so the soul can leave or it may be required that only a family member can touch the body*)

- Should anyone in particular be informed about your death (*this can be very important when there are any family conflicts e.g. two sets of children because of divorce and remarriages*)
- What do you want to happen to your physical remains? (*some people may want to donate organs to help other people or to donate their body for medical research*)
- Do you want to be buried or cremated?
- Do you have any specific requests regarding:

  - Type of coffin
  - Clothing: how you want to be dressed
  - Jewellery: to be worn
  - Anything to be placed in the coffin

- Do you want a funeral service or some other type of ceremony? If yes:

  - Where should this take place? (*e.g. church, crematorium, elsewhere*)
  - Who should conduct the service/ceremony?
  - Who should be invited to attend?
  - Should anyone not attend?
  - What do you want to happen during the service/ceremony? (*e.g. hymns/ songs/tunes; speakers/musicians/actors; readings/poetry/anecdotes*)
  - Do you want flowers?
  - Do you want donations to be made? (*e.g. to specific organisations, charities*)
  - Place for burial (*e.g. cemetery; woodland burial; specific plot*)
  - Location for cremation.
  - Are there any particular words, pictures, symbols that should be on a headstone/plaque?
  - If cremated, what should be done with the ashes?

- Should there be a wake/party after the service?
- Is there anything else you need to do in preparation for your eventual death?

Print name:
Signature:
Date:
Time:

25 Man in the corner

Introduction

When I worked in a children's hospital at the beginning of my social work career, I spent a lot of time with children who were dying; many of them had been diagnosed with leukaemia, other forms of cancer or had brain tumours. I spent a lot of my time talking to children of all ages about their pending death. Most of their concerns were for their parents rather than themselves. A commonality was that many of the children would see a man in the corner of the room before passing away. The child would often say that the man had taken them to 'heaven' to see what it was like and that it was 'alright'. S/he would then reassure the parents that it was all going to be fine and they had nothing to worry about. The child would be able to describe exactly what they had seen and done with the man in the corner. After having this experience, the child often passed over quite quickly i.e. within a day or two. There were many discussions amongst social workers, nurses and doctors whether this was a spiritual experience or due to the medication. There were lots of different opinions and viewpoints.

I wrote the following script many years later as a hypnotherapist, because my own image of the man in the corner had always stayed with me. The image of the man had developed from how he had been described by so many different children. It was written for a child of any age and the child does not have to have any religious beliefs or believe there is a heaven. The objective is for the child to imagine and experience the feeling of being peaceful and not afraid. However, there is no reason why it could not be used for an adult who does have religious or spiritual beliefs. I wrote the script so it could be read to a child, but the hypnotherapist may choose to ask questions once the child has gone through the corner in the room and is on the other side in order to find out what s/he is seeing.

When working with young children I tend to use the term 'special mind' when referring to the subconscious. This term is used in the script but the hypnotherapist may replace it with their own terminology or what the child prefers to use.

DOI: 10.4324/9781032245706-28

The script

I just want you to close your eyes and shut out the rest of the world. You know how to do this now – how to relax and go anywhere you want. I know you have been feeling *(insert as appropriate to the child: tired; in pain; wanting it all to be over or any other specific things which may have been talked about)*. It would be so good for you to imagine feeling relaxed so you can become even more relaxed – and for you to feel calm – having nothing to worry about. It is only natural to worry about things we know little or nothing about. Sometimes we need someone to help us and show us the way.

So take some gentle breaths in and out. Breathe in now very gently – and now breathe out even more gently. That's right – and again. Breathe in very gently – and now breathe out even more gently. That's good. You are relaxing more and more. And again – breathe in very gently – and now breathe out even more gently. Well done. Continue to breathe gently – very gently. As you continue to breathe gently you feel more and more relaxed and calm. Now I am going to ask you to imagine certain things, because I know you are very good at using your special mind.

Imagine now you are looking into one of the corners of the room. Focus your attention completely on the corner you have chosen in the room. Imagine that the corner of the room is completely empty – there is no furniture in it – nothing on the floor – it is completely empty. Keep looking at that empty corner in the room. Look at the corner – from the top where it reaches into the ceiling – down to the bottom where it reaches into the floor. You know something is about to appear – just wait – keep watching the corner. Suddenly a man walks out of the corner. A gentle and kind man – someone who has come to help you. Someone you can trust – someone who can answer any questions you might have. You can talk to the gentle and kind man about anything.

The gentle and kind man is standing in the corner. I wonder what he looks like. Look at him. I wonder whether:

- He is young or old
- He is short or tall
- His hair is short or long.

(Guidance note: the hypnotherapist can choose to ask the child to describe the man or ask specific questions to get more detail)

What I do know is the man in the corner is gentle and kind. Look at the man's face – he is smiling at you. He is stretching both of his arms out to you. He is beckoning to you. He is going to show you a very beautiful place – a place where you can rest and be peaceful. Go with the gentle and kind man. Walk towards the corner in the room – follow the gentle and kind man. Now go through the corner in the wall – follow the gentle and kind man.

Keep following the gentle and kind man. You can trust him. You feel safe being with him. You can ask him anything you want. As you follow the gentle and kind man – you feel more and more at peace. Nothing bothers you at all. You just feel peaceful. Enjoy walking with the gentle and kind man in this beautiful place. Look around you – I wonder what you see. Walk with the gentle and kind man – explore this beautiful peaceful place. Talk to the gentle and kind man. Talk to the gentle and kind man about this place. Ask him about it. Talk to the gentle and kind man about how you feel. Ask him about anything – things you want to know. He will talk to you – he will be honest with you – he will help you in any way he can. He is a gentle and kind man.

(Guidance note: if the hypnotherapist does want to ask direct questions and get responses from the child the following questions can be used)

What are you seeing *(or sensing if the child is not visual)* exactly?
What is it like in this place?
How are you feeling?
What do you want to do?
Where do you want to go?
Is the gentle and kind man saying anything to you?
Do you want to ask the gentle and kind man anything?

So stay with the gentle and kind man for as long as you like. Enjoy feeling peaceful. You know there is nothing to be scared of here in this beautiful place. Nothing bothers you at all. You just feel peaceful. Enjoy being with the gentle and kind man in this beautiful peaceful place.

26 Animal heaven

Introduction

It is generally thought that a child starts to understand the concept of death from the age of six. Before then they will still miss a person or animal that has died, but may not be able to understand that the person/animal is never coming back. They still need to grieve for that person/animal and be able to talk about them. As a hypnotherapist I work with children from the age of five upwards and believe that death needs to be talked about when a death occurs and a child should be encouraged to grieve. I wrote the script below specifically for a young child who has lost an animal, which may be the first bereavement s/he will experience. There is a short introduction at the beginning of the script to bring in the subject of the animal and suggests the animal is now living somewhere else. The hypnotherapist will discover where the animal is living and then use one of the four alternative locations (farm; circus, zoo or any other place the child mentions) to visit the animal. Eventually the idea is embedded that the animal will continue to live elsewhere and will not be coming back.

Other scripts to help children with bereavement can be found in Chapter 24 of *'Hypnotherapy Scripts to Promote Children's Wellbeing'*.[1]

The script

I know you are really sad because *(insert name of animal)* is no longer living with you. I know you are going to miss him/her and it will feel strange not having him/her around. I am sure s/he is going to miss you too. When you are feeling very sad, it can help a bit if you try to think happy thoughts. Think about things you and *(name of animal)* did together – you will never forget those happy times. *(Name of animal)* has gone to be somewhere else now – somewhere where they can live, play, sleep – and most importantly be happy. I wonder if you can imagine where that might be. You know that your special mind can take you anywhere. Think about where *(name of animal)* would be very happy to live in the future – a farm – a circus – a zoo – or somewhere else maybe. Think about what

DOI: 10.4324/9781032245706-29

(name of animal) might like to do to have some fun. Think about where *(name of animal)* could make some new friends. Perhaps a farm – a circus – a zoo – or somewhere else. Where do you think *(name of animal)* will be? *(await response)*. So imagine what *(name of animal)* is doing right now in *(location named by the child)*.

(Guidance note: depending on how the child responds the hypnotherapist will use one of the scripts below followed by the questions)

Location 1: Farm

Just imagine you are arriving on the farm where *(name of animal)* now lives. You are standing in the farmyard. You will see the farmhouse where the farmer and his family live. There are probably some other buildings as well where the farm workers live and sleep. Look at which animals you can see walking around the farmyard – chickens – hens – ducks – dogs – cats. I wonder if you can hear any noises – hens clucking – dogs barking – cats meowing – ducks quacking around the pond – cows mooing in the fields – horses neighing in the stables – birds singing. A farm is a very busy place. There are lots of comings and goings – as well as the animals and humans there may be cars – tractors – so much going on outdoors and indoors.

I wonder where *(name of animal)* might be. Why don't you have a look around the farm – the farmhouse – the farmyard – the barns – the stables – the fields? I wonder where s/he might be. Go and find him/her now and tell me when you see him/her.

Oh fantastic. Tell me what *(name of animal)* is doing.

How does *(name of animal)* look?

Does *(name of animal)* look happy?

Ask *(name of animal)* to show you around the farm.

Would you like to see where *(name of animal)* is living now? *(e.g. where s/he eats/sleeps)*

Ask *(name of animal)* to introduce you to some of the other animals.

What else would you like to see on the farm?

Would you like to spend some time playing with *(name of animal)*?

Is there anything else you would like to do with *(name of animal)*?

Is there anything you would like to ask *(name of animal)*?

Is there anything you would like to tell *(name of animal)*?

Is there anything else you would like to talk about with *(name of animal)*?

Location 2: Circus

You are arriving at the circus. You can see the big top where all the exciting acts will perform. Imagine all the people in their seats – eagerly waiting for the entertainment to begin. The ring master is standing at the place where the performers run into the ring. The clowns are walking round the outside of the ring with their painted faces – funny clothes and big feet. I wonder who will be performing today – what you might see. The tightrope walkers can walk so confidently across the wire. The trapeze artists can climb high up ropes then swing across the air. There could be jugglers – magicians – dancers – musicians – cyclists – all sorts of entertainment for you to enjoy.

Which act do you think *(name of animal)* would like to watch? I wonder where s/he is. Outside the big top there are lots of eating places – amusements – caravans where the performers live, sleep and get ready for their performance. Why not have a wander around and see if you can find *(name of animal)* – see what s/he is doing? Tell me when you find him/her.

Oh fantastic. Tell me what *(name of animal)* is doing.

How does *(name of animal)* look?

Does *(name of animal)* look happy?

Ask *(name of animal)* to show you around the circus.

Would you like to see where *(name of animal)* is living now? *(e.g. where s/he eats/sleeps)*

Would you like to meet anyone else who lives at the circus?

Would you like to spend some time playing with *(name of animal)* before the performance begins?

Is there anything else you would like to do with (*name of animal)* before the performance begins?

Is there anything you would like to ask *(name of animal)* before the performance begins?

Is there anything you would like to tell *(name of animal)* before the performance begins?

Is there anything else you would like to talk about with *(name of animal)* before the performance begins?

Would you like to go into the big top now and watch some of the acts with *(name of animal)*?

Location 3: Zoo

You have come to the zoo to find *(name of animal)*. It will be fun to find where *(name of animal)* is living exactly in the zoo and what s/he has been doing since getting here. So go through the entrance and start wandering around the zoo. There are so many different animals living here. It might take some time to walk round all the different places. I wonder what you might see first. Maybe some big animals in cages – lions – tigers – cheetahs – gorillas. Or animals in large open spaces outside the buildings where they sleep – elephants – camels – giraffes – bears – rhinoceroses – hippopotamuses. The smaller animals may be in the reptile house – or the butterfly house. There are so many birds to see – both big and small – in the birdhouse. So where do you think *(name of animal)* might be hanging out? Who do you think s/he would play with – make friends with? Go and see if you can find *(name of animal)*. Tell me when you have found him/her.

Oh fantastic. Tell me what *(name of animal)* is doing.
How does *(name of animal)* look?
Ask *(name of animal)* to show you around the zoo.
Does *(name of animal)* look happy?
Would you like to see where *(name of animal)* is living now? *(e.g. where s/he eats/sleeps)*
Ask *(name of animal)* to introduce you to some of the other animals.
Is there anything else you would like to see at the zoo?
Would you like to spend some time playing with *(name of animal)*?
Is there anything else you would like to do with *(name of animal)?*
Is there anything you would like to ask *(name of animal)?*
Is there anything you would like to tell *(name of animal)?*
Is there anything else you would like to talk about with *(name of animal)?*

Location 4: Any other place

So as you are imagining *(name of animal)*, tell me where s/he is now. Oh that is good that *(name of animal)* has found a new place to live. Tell me more about this place.

What is it like?
What do you see?
How does *(name of animal)* look?
Does *(name of animal)* look happy?
What is *(name of animal)* doing?
Ask *(name of animal)* to show you around.
Where does *(name of animal)* eat?
Where does *(name of animal)* sleep?
Ask *(name of animal)* who s/he plays with?
Would you like to spend some time playing with *(name of animal)*?
Is there anything else you would like to do with *(name of animal)?*
Is there anything else you would like to ask *(name the animal)?*
Is there anything you would like to tell *(name of animal)?*
Is there anything else you would like to talk about with *(name of animal)?*

Ending for all locations

That was good wasn't it – your special mind taking you to see and play with *(name of animal)*? It is good to know that *(name of animal)* has found somewhere new to live now s/he cannot live with you. It is good to know that *(name of animal)* is happy, well and safe in his/her new home with new friends. *(Name of animal)* will never forget you, just like you will never forget him/her. And any time you want to see or play with *(name of animal)* you just have to use your special mind to take you to *(insert farm, circus, zoo or other location)*.

Note

1 Pritchard, J. (2021) *Hypnotherapy Scripts to Promote Children's Wellbeing.* Abingdon, Oxon: Routledge.

27 Conversations on the clouds

Introduction

One of the most common subjects to be discussed when working with a bereaved person is regrets. However, when a person experiences any type of loss they may regret that they did not say or do something. I originally wrote this script for a bereaved person, but have found it useful for anyone who needs to work on their regrets after experiencing a loss. The script can also be used to rehearse conversations when someone needs to get answers from another person (e.g. when they have been passed over for promotion or been made redundant), but they are dreading having the conversation; or they feel very unconfident about confronting the person.

The beginning of the script can be used as an introduction to trance and a deepener. Some clients choose to have the clouds as their safe place and return there purely for relaxation purposes.

The script

I want you to imagine that you are travelling on an aeroplane. You have a window seat and no-one is sitting next to you, so you can spread out as much as you like. Stretch your arms and legs out as far as you like and relax. Just make yourself really comfortable. Start to feel really relaxed. Feel that relaxation starting to move from the top of your head as it leans against the headrest. Feel the relaxation moving down your arms and into your hands. The relaxation is moving down the front of your body – and then down the back of you as you relax more into the back of the seat. Relaxing more and more now. Feel the relaxation moving down and down – down into your legs and into your feet. You are sinking further down into the seat. Really relaxed now.

There are other passengers in the cabin, but just let the different noises you might be hearing fade into the background. You might hear some people talking – the squeak of the wheels on the flight attendant's trolley – music coming out of someone's headphones – the aeroplane's engine – the pilot's voice giving a message. Just let any noises fade into the

DOI: 10.4324/9781032245706-30

background – fade right away – so you hear nothing at all – nothing bothers you at all. You are experiencing total peace and quiet. That's right – total peace and quiet.

As you are feeling so peaceful, so quiet and so relaxed, just look out of the window. You can see the sky. I wonder what colour it is today. You also see lots of fluffy, brilliant white clouds. There are so many of them – all different shapes and sizes – but all of them are very fluffy and brilliant white. Just start to look at some of the clouds that are nearest to the window. Look at the different shapes. Look at the different shades of white in each one. Now look further into the distance – see more fluffy, brilliant white clouds. Look at the different shapes. Look at the different shades of white in each one.

There are so many fluffy, brilliant white clouds. They almost look like a brilliant, white blanket strewn across the sky. I wonder how many clouds you can actually see. Why don't you start counting them? Start counting the clouds nearest to the window – *1, 2, 3, 4, 5* – keep counting *(pause)*. Keep counting – counting the clouds in the distance – keep counting *(pause)*.

It can be so relaxing counting the clouds – watching the clouds. Some clouds might seem like they are not moving at all – they are static. Others might be moving – some slowly – some quickly. First watch the stillness. Then watch the movement. The clouds that are static know their place – they have come to rest – they are so calming. The clouds that are moving all have a purpose – they are on a journey – they know where they want to go and what they need to do.

All the fluffy, brilliant white clouds look very comfortable. You can just imagine how you might sink down into a cloud – feeling safe and secure. All the fluffy, brilliant white clouds can serve lots of different purposes. They can help you relax by making you feel very comfortable, but they can also be good places to have conversations. You can always talk to yourself – talk to your subconscious mind – it will always give you the right answers. The fluffy, brilliant white clouds can also bring people to talk to you. You can ask the clouds to bring people to talk to you.

(Guidance note: at this point the hypnotherapist can choose to do some more relaxation work using the clouds and creating them as a safe place for the client before moving on to the rest of the script)

I know you have been feeling *(sad, upset, angry, regretful or any other emotion discussed with the client previously)* and it might be helpful to talk about some of the things you have been feeling or to say some of the things you regret that you never said to someone *(or insert a specific person if appropriate)*.

It is time to stand up and get out of your seat on the aeroplane – move into the aisle. Look around for the nearest exit – look for a door that will open.

When you see it, make your way towards it. Stand in front of the door – you are feeling calm. Take some deep breaths – in and out – in and out – that's right. Now look for the handle on the door – see which way you need to turn it to open the door. On the count of *3*, you will open the door – *1, 2, and 3*. Do not go through the doorway just yet. Just put your head outside and have a good look around. Look at all the fluffy, brilliant white clouds. So many clouds – all different shapes and sizes. Decide which cloud you would like to stand or sit on. I wonder if it will be one nearby or one in the far distance. You choose. When you have chosen your cloud you will feel ready to leave the aeroplane.

On the count of *3*, you are going to leave the aeroplane and you can either – step, hop, skip, jump or fly onto the cloud you have chosen. Ready now – *1, 2, and 3*. Out you go and onto the cloud. Make yourself comfortable on the cloud. Just sink right down into it – feeling safe and supported. That's right – safe and supported. You need to know that you can make the cloud travel if you want to do so – you can just tell it to travel in the right direction – it will know where to go. Or you can just stay where you are – the cloud will remain static.

Now it is time to have a conversation with *(name of person)*. Just start thinking about *(name of person)*. Perhaps you want to remember what s/he looked like. Or maybe you might be thinking about times you spent together – things that were said – things that were not said. Think about things you would like to say to *(name of person)*. While you are thinking your cloud can start to move or it can remain static – it really does not matter – you choose what you want the cloud to do. Just keep thinking about *(name of person)*. Look into the distance. Look at all the fluffy, brilliant white clouds surrounding you and in the far distance. Keep looking – keep looking. Soon you are going to see *(name of person)* on a cloud coming towards you. Keep thinking about what you want to talk about because you are going to have a conversation with *(name of person)*. A conversation on the clouds.

It is important that you say what you need to say. Ask any questions that you need to ask.

(Guidance note: the hypnotherapist will work with the client whilst they have the conversation with the person. After the conversation has been completed another person can be brought in on another cloud if needed or the clouds can be returned to in another session)

So now you have finished your conversation(s), take some time to just relax on the cloud. Sink really deep down into the cloud – relax – feel good that you have been able to have a conversation. Just relax now – let your mind drift – stay on the cloud as long as you need to do so.

28 The great pyramid

Introduction

This chapter is concerned with remembering and commemorating. It contains the main script which is an introduction and deepener; followed by three additional scripts which will facilitate remembering, commemorating and talking to a deceased person.

Just like people react differently to a death and how they cope with that loss, people will have different views on how someone should be remembered or commemorated – if at all. In recent years, I have worked with a number of teenagers and young adults who have been bereaved and yet had not realised the impact this had had on their lives and how it was affecting their current behaviours. Because I like to find the root cause of a problem when I am working with any client, bereavement has come to light when working with these young people. Another commonality has been that parents or other relatives have refused to talk about the deceased person or they have been told it is 'not a good idea' or 'it would not be good for you' to visit the cemetery where the person is buried. In my practice I encourage clients to remember and commemorate a person they have lost.

Through visiting the great pyramid a bereaved person can go into trance and then spend time exploring and relaxing. Additional script 1 is specifically for remembering a deceased person. Additional script 2 facilitates commemorating the deceased person. The objective of additional script 3 is to meet the deceased person and be able to work on any unresolved issues.

The script

Right in front of you there is a camel sitting on the ground. It is waiting for you to climb on its back and go on a journey. When you are ready – approach the camel – and climb onto the seat that is on the camel's back. Get yourself settled on the camel and take hold of the reins. Then sit very still and wait for the camel to rise onto its feet. As the camel starts to

DOI: 10.4324/9781032245706-31

stand up you start to feel excited – wondering where the camel is going to take you. The camel starts to walk forward – you feel safe as the camel transports you. It is a smooth journey – not bumpy at all. You feel very safe on top of the camel.

You and the camel are going across fine, yellow sand – you realise you are in a desert. The sun is beating down – it is a hot, dry day. There is a water bottle hanging down on the side of the camel – take a drink whenever you need it. The camel continues to walk smoothly – elegantly across the desert. Enjoy the journey – look around you. Above is a clear blue sky – below you is the fine, yellow sand which stretches for miles and miles across the desert.

As you are enjoying travelling on the camel, keep looking into the distance. There may be nothing in particular to see at the moment – just enjoy the journey. Feeling safe and calm. Look into the distance again and you see something. It is something that appears to be very small – but you are aware that it is wide at the bottom but has a sharp point at the top. The camel continues to take you forward on the journey – getting closer to the shape you are seeing in the distance – closer and closer. As you get nearer you realise you are looking at a pyramid. As you get closer and closer, the pyramid seems to get bigger and bigger. Closer and closer now. You are amazed how big and magnificent the pyramid is. Closer and closer – and then you are there – right at the entrance. The camel stops and then moves downwards to sit on the ground. It is time for you to dismount from the camel.

A pyramid is a place where a person can rest in peace after they have lived their life on earth. Many Egyptian kings and queens had their pyramids built during their own lifetimes – building the outside and inside of their pyramid just as they wanted it to be. A place where they could rest – be at peace – and also have all their important possessions and treasures with them forever. Now the pyramid you are standing in front of belongs to *(deceased person)*. The pyramid is a place where you can come to see *(deceased person)* – talk with *(deceased person)* – or you can just sit quietly in the pyramid and think about *(deceased person)* – remember him/her.

It is time now to go into the pyramid and explore all the different places within it. The rooms in a pyramid are known as chambers and there will be many corridors and tunnels going up and down inside the pyramid. It will be exciting to explore inside the pyramid and see what you find. So on the count of *3*, go into the pyramid – *1, 2,* and *3.* Go through the entrance and into the pyramid. As you leave the sunlight and brightness behind you, you enter into darkness. Your eyes gradually get used to the darkness – you can see in front of you. You then realise there are some candles or lanterns on the walls which are lighting up the corridor in front of you, so you can walk forward with confidence.

Look around you – see the walls – made of huge blocks of stone. I wonder if anything is written or drawn on the walls. Choose which direction you would like to go in. You will see that there are corridors leading off the corridor you are walking along. There are also steps leading down to tunnels, which go down deep into the lower levels of the pyramid. Go in whichever direction want – keep walking. Go into any chamber that you want to explore – see what treasures you can find. You may see drawings – pictures – statues.

(Guidance note: the hypnotherapist should then spend some time exploring the pyramid with the client before proceeding to meet the deceased person. However, sometimes the deceased person appears suddenly during the exploration. If this happens go straight to additional script 3)

You have had a good look around the pyramid – you know where everything is – so you can come back any time you like and use the chambers. Now it is time to think about *(deceased person)*. Let your mind drift back to some happy memories.

(Guidance note: the hypnotherapist can then decide how they want to work with the client and use the additional scripts as and when required)

Additional script 1: Remembering

You have explored the pyramid now – you know where the corridors and tunnels lead to – you know there are lots of different chambers. The pyramid is a place where you can return to any time you like just to sit and think about *(deceased person)*. It is a quiet, peaceful place – somewhere you can be alone with your thoughts and memories. When someone you care about dies, you can experience all sorts of emotions and at times you may feel that you cannot cope – you cannot go on. When you feel lost and do not know what to do, it can help to go deep into the pyramid and spend time remembering – your memories will never die – they will always be within you. Memories can be a comfort. You may find things in the chambers that remind you of *(deceased person)* because a pyramid stores possessions and treasures from life on earth. You might also find things which *(deceased person)* is using in his/her new life.

Start walking around the pyramid again and find a chamber you want to go in to remember *(deceased person)*. Tell me when you have found that chamber. Go into the chamber now and tell me what you see. Find somewhere to sit in the chamber. Make yourself comfortable – close your eyes – and let your memories of *(deceased person)* drift into your mind. There is no need to force anything – just let the memories drift into your mind. Remember *(deceased person)* – let the memories drift into your mind – drift – and remember *(deceased person)*. Tell me about *(deceased person)*.

(Guidance note: the hypnotherapist should let the client talk and remember for as long as they need to do so)

Maybe you would like to look around this chamber and see what you can find. Or maybe you would like to go into another chamber. What would you like to do?

(Guidance note: the hypnotherapist should wait for the client to decide before proceeding further in the current chamber or going to another chamber)

OK so now explore the chamber. The chamber will be storing important objects, which will help you remember *(deceased person)* – and bring forward more memories. These objects will help you remember *(deceased person)*. Keep looking until you find an object. Tell me what you have found. Sit with and hold/look at *(object)* – what does it bring into your mind? What are you remembering?

(Guidance note: the hypnotherapist should discuss what is being remembered. More memories can be brought forward by looking at more objects in the chamber)

Additional script 2: Commemorating

You are sitting in one of the chambers of the pyramid. You are relaxing – breathing nice and steadily – relaxing more and more. When you are deeply relaxed physically your mind relaxes too and you can see things more clearly. Today you are going to think about how you can commemorate *(deceased person)*. You know you can remember *(deceased person)* any time you wish to do so. You can visualise *(deceased person)* – recall a memory – a particular time or experience – you can relive a feeling. Remembering is good, but it can also be helpful to commemorate a person – do something to celebrate their life – what they did – what they achieved. Some people choose to commemorate a person on a particular day or at a particular time. It really does not matter when or how it is done. People have their own way of commemorating – planting a tree – placing flowers on a grave – putting a plaque on a wall or bench – releasing a balloon – lighting a candle. There are so many ways to commemorate a person. As you are sitting so comfortably now – thinking about *(deceased person)* – keep relaxing – and think about how you would like to commemorate *(deceased person)*. You will know the best way to do this. Just relax – and think about how you would like to commemorate *(deceased person)*. Take your time.

(Guidance note: the hypnotherapist will then work with the client to get the detail regarding the commemoration. The following questions can be used if required)

How are you going to commemorate *(deceased person)*?
What will you do exactly?
When will you do this? *(e.g. on a specific day/date; time)*
How often will you do this? *(being mindful the client may only choose to do this once)*

Where will you do this?
Will you do this with anyone else?

Additional script 3: Meeting the deceased person

There is one particular chamber in the pyramid where *(deceased person)* will like to rest and sleep. Find that chamber now – when you have found it just stand outside for a moment. You are about to meet *(deceased person)* s/he is waiting for you. Now go into the chamber and there *(deceased person)* is.

How is s/he looking?
What is s/he wearing?
What else do you see in the chamber?
Go forward and greet *(deceased person)*. You can now spend some time with *(deceased person)*.

(Guidance note: the hypnotherapist should use the following prompts as appropriate to help the client talk to the deceased person and focus on/ resolve any particular questions/issues/concerns)

This is the time for you to:

Tell *(deceased person)* how you have been feeling.
Explain how their death has affected you.
Articulate anything that you need to discuss (and did not or could not say before the death occurred).
Find out what happened (e.g. in regard to the death or any other matter that is important to you).

Ask any questions you may have:

About the death
The reason for doing what s/he did (e.g. suicide)
The reason for saying/doing related to something from the past
The reason for not saying/doing related to something from the past
How *(deceased person)* has been since passing over/in the pyramid
How *(deceased person)* is now.

You have had a good conversation with *(deceased person)*. You have discussed what you needed to and you have seen that *(deceased person)* is resting and at peace *(and insert anything else positive that has come out during the meeting)*. Let your own mind find some peace now. You have been grieving and experiencing so many emotions – and you still have more things to face in the future – but you can do that knowing *(deceased person)* is fine and you can come back to the pyramid at any time and talk to him/her again.

29 The storage unit

Introduction

This is another script to facilitate remembering a person. The previous chapter presented scripts which focussed on working with bereavement. The script in this chapter can be used for a bereaved client, but I wrote it originally for any client who needed to remember the positive things about a person and/or relationship when it has ended. Since writing the original version and using it for a specific purpose, I have on occasions used it to retrieve some good memories for the client from their life in general – perhaps when they are feeling low for some unknown reason and they need a bit of a boost i.e. remembering that their life has not always been gloomy.

The script can also be used to facilitate regression work. I have found that sometimes when using this script a bad memory (or memories) can come forward and work needs to be undertaken to work through the associated negative thoughts and feelings. Once the storage unit has been created, it can be returned to in future sessions to work on specific memories/past events and to use regression techniques. Of course the client should be encouraged to use it themselves at any time they feel the need to recall a positive memory.

The script

Your subconscious mind will always carry your memories. Everything is stored safely in your subconscious mind. It can be good to work with your subconscious mind to create special ways of remembering things or celebrating something. People sometimes go out of our lives and there is nothing that we can do to bring them back. It is so important to try to remember the good things about the person – the good things about the relationship – the positive things that happened – the happy memories – rather than focussing on the negatives. I want you to start thinking about (*person/relationship*).

You are standing on a very busy road. Traffic is flowing in both directions on the actual road and people are hurrying along the pavements. It

DOI: 10.4324/9781032245706-32

feels like a very busy day. You need to take some time out to relax and remember. You need to get away from this busy-ness. Look around you and you will see the outside of one of those storage places – where people put their belongings in a unit for safe keeping. It is a huge building that you see. There is a sign on the building: 'Safe Storage: Store Your Memories Here'. Walk towards the building and find the entrance to it. There will be a car park for lorries – removal vans – smaller vans – cars – motorbikes – bicycles. All sorts of people use this storage place – people moving house – business people – sales people – couriers – students. They all have their reasons for storing things. Somewhere there will be a door to the reception area. You need to go into the reception area and collect a master key, so you can find yourself a suitable unit. A person in the reception area gives you a key and points you in the direction of a lift.

This storage place has many floors and lots of different sized units on each floor. You need to find the one that is right for you. You need to find a unit where you can store your memories of *(person/relationship)* and where you can come to just sit and remember. A perfect place just for you and your memories. Walk towards the lift and press the call button. When the doors open step in and choose which floor you would like to go to. As the doors close push the button to go to the floor you have chosen. The lift travels gently and smoothly to the floor you have chosen. When the doors open again step out and you find yourself on a corridor. There are lots of corridors on this floor going in many directions – and units all of different sizes. Start exploring now – go along the corridors. You have the master key so you can go into any unit to have a look around. Take your time – look in as many units as you like. It is important to find the right sized unit for you. Tell me what you see as you walk along the corridors and look in the units.

(Guidance note: the hypnotherapist should work with the client as s/he explores the units. Some questions and prompts are listed below for use if required)

Where are you now?
What is this unit like?
How does it feel being in this unit?
Is this the right unit for you and your memories?
If it does not feel right come out of that unit, shut the door and lock up the unit.
Go and find another unit – the right one for you.

(Guidance note: the questions above can be repeated as many times as needed until the client finds the right unit)

Great you have found the right storage unit for you. You have a lot of memories to bring into the unit. I wonder how you are going to store them. Do you need any shelves – bookcases – filing cabinets – storage boxes? What would you like to have in your unit? You are going to spend time in here remembering. So do you need to bring in some furniture – a chair – a table? Maybe some food or drink – or even a fridge? Whatever you need, bring those things in now.

(Guidance note: the hypnotherapist should prompt the client to find out what is happening/being brought in)

So your storage unit is ready for your memories. Sit or lie down – make yourself comfortable in your storage unit. It is time to remember. Start bringing memories of *(person/relationship)* forward. Tell me about each individual memory as it comes forward.

(Guidance note: the hypnotherapist explores each memory with the client. Not all memories that come forward will be good/positive and some work may be needed to release the associated negative feeling(s). It is at this point that the hypnotherapist may wish to do some regression work. Where there is a good memory the client should relive it and then store it somewhere in the unit)

That is such a good memory. Where would you like to store it – to keep it safe? OK – put it away now. Would you like to bring forward another memory for remembering and storage?

(Guidance note: the hypnotherapist continues until the client is ready to stop remembering and storing memories)

You have done really well in bringing forward memories today. You can come back to your storage unit at any time to remember *(person/relationship)*. Of course you can think about *(person/relationship)* any time you like – wherever you are – but it is good to take time out and have a place where you can really concentrate on remembering. It helps to bring forward your memories of *(person/relationship)* and remember. *(Person/relationship)* will always live on in your thoughts and in your heart. Many memories will be stored but you may not always remember all of them in the conscious state. You can come back to your storage unit at any time and bring forward lots of memories which are hidden in your subconscious mind. Enjoy being in your storage unit and remembering *(person/relationship)*. For now though, close the door to your unit and lock it up, so that all your memories are safe and secure.

30 The red admiral butterfly

Introduction

There are many people who believe that there is no existence after life on earth. Others who have religious or spiritual beliefs would tend to disagree – they believe something does happen or exist after life. Some people believe in reincarnation – that we come back to live another life. It is important for the hypnotherapist when undertaking an assessment with a client who has been bereaved, to discuss the client's beliefs before starting any therapy with them. The hypnotherapist needs a clear understanding about any beliefs a client may have – whether they be religious, spiritual or something else. In many texts written about death and bereavement, attention is given to the fact that many people imagine seeing, hearing the person they are grieving for. Some clients may believe that a dead person can come back in the form of an animal. The following script is metaphorical and I have found it helps and gives comfort to clients who question their own beliefs or senses having experienced a bereavement.

The script

I want to tell you about a woman called Lydia and the red butterfly. I think imagining Lydia and the red butterfly might help you. Lydia was considered to be a strong, intelligent, coping woman. After her husband Gus died, very suddenly and unexpectedly, she was distraught as they had been together a long time.

One day in May, Lydia was sitting reading in her garden. She looked up and saw a beautiful red and black butterfly. It flew onto one of the rose bushes in the garden. Lydia looked closely at the butterfly. Its wings were basically black with red lines and odd little white bits – looking like they had been splashed on. It was a red admiral butterfly. Can you imagine what it looked like? Lydia was fascinated by the butterfly. She loved butterflies anyway but she felt particularly drawn to this one. The butterfly stayed on the rose bush for quite a long time and Lydia never took her eyes off it. She kept looking at the markings on the butterfly's wings.

DOI: 10.4324/9781032245706-33

The next day was another nice day, so Lydia went out in the garden again to read. The butterfly appeared again as soon as she had got herself settled in the chair. The butterfly flew around the garden for a while and then settled on the rose bush. For a second time it stayed for quite a while. Lydia once again studied closely the markings on the butterfly's black wings – the red lines and odd little white bits. The butterfly returned regularly through the summer months – it appeared every time Lydia was in the garden. Lydia knew it was the same butterfly because of the markings on its wings.

Lydia was a working woman who had her own business which she ran in an office in the city centre. She travelled a lot with work so was not in the office every day. One day she was in the office and it was very, very hot, so she opened the window and suddenly the red and black butterfly flew in. She just knew by the markings on the wings, it was the same butterfly who visited her garden. Black wings with the red lines and odd little white bits – the markings were exactly the same. She felt a sense of familiarity. The butterfly flew onto one of the bookcases and stayed there. The butterfly then became a regular visitor to both the garden and the office.

Lydia truly believed the butterfly was Gus. Whenever it was around she felt less sad, more at peace and she talked to the butterfly. Most of her friends said she was imagining it all and 'she'd get over it'. Once the summer had ended, Lydia did not see the butterfly as often and by the autumn she did not see it at all. Butterflies do not live very long so she concluded it was dead.

At Christmas, Lydia decided to go abroad for the holidays so she did not have to think about previous Christmases spent with Gus. She loved going to hot climates, to relax on a beach and do virtually nothing. The first day she walked down to the beach she found a nice quiet spot and was just putting the towel on the sun lounger when a red and black butterfly flew out of her bag. She just knew by the markings on the wings, it was the same butterfly who had visited her garden and the office. Black wings with the red lines and odd little white bits – the markings were exactly the same. She felt a sense of familiarity. She knew that Gus had come on holiday with her.

Lydia felt at peace whenever she saw the butterfly and she got great comfort from having the butterfly around her. She talked to the butterfly – shared things she could tell no-one else Whether or not you believe it was Gus is not important. Everyone has their own beliefs regarding whether something happens after life here on earth or not. The butterfly was an important part of Lydia's life and it helped her while she grieved for Gus. However, you choose to deal with your grief is absolutely fine – you have to do what is right for you. If you believe a person you have lost comes back to you or is around you in a different form – as a living thing – a spirit – or some form of energy – then take comfort from that and grieve how you need to do so.

Part IV
Moving forward

31 Acceptance and aspirations

Introduction

One of the main objectives in grief work for any therapist is to help the client to work towards accepting whatever loss they have experienced. Acceptance is one of the final stages of any journey of grief, no matter what theory or model of grief is being used. Part IV in this book is focussed on looking to the future and in hypnotherapy terms 'forward pacing'. The first chapter in the section contains a script to introduce the client to the concept of acceptance. Much of the work will have been done at this stage and the treatment plan nearing completion. The hypnotherapist should use the acceptance script below and then choose scripts from the other chapters in Part IV to help the client look to the future and plan.

Appendix 31.1 consists of three sections to help focus on the client's aspirations. Section A contains a list of questions which are used in the main script. Section B can be used to list the client's aspirations. Section C is for developing an Aspirations Plan. The hypnotherapist can use the appendix to make notes during a session and it can also be used for more in-depth recording after a session has taken place. The aspiration list and aspiration plan can be typed up after a session and given to the client.

The script

I want to congratulate you on the way you have been working through your journey of grief. Such a journey is never easy – there are a lot of ups and downs – going forwards and backwards – maybe lots of turns. It is easy to lose your way at times on such a journey. You have been doing so well in these sessions – exploring and working through your emotions. It is now time to think about acceptance and what that means to you. Once you have accepted something you can move forward and face the future. You cannot change what has happened in the past but you can change how you think and feel about it. I think you are at the stage now where

DOI: 10.4324/9781032245706-35

you have done that. Let's get you to look at the progress you have made since you experienced *(the loss)* and started on your journey of grief. I want you to focus on the positives – what you have learnt and what you have achieved.

You are just going to let your mind drift back to when we first met and you came to work through your loss and grief. Can you visualise yourself walking into the therapy room? Remember how you were. You might want to do this by looking from a distance – there is no need to relive any pain you were experiencing then – you have done that already. Just look from afar – look how you were. Drift back a little further – look how you were when you first experienced the loss. It was hard to believe what had happened – disbelief – some denial *(insert any other reaction the client had to the loss at the time)*. It was such a difficult time – but you got through it – and since then you have worked through the loss and your grief. Remember to focus on the positives – what you have learnt and what you have achieved. Keep looking back at yourself – your journey of grief – your progress. Now tell me about the positives you remember from being on your journey of grief. What do you see looking back? What do you remember? What have you learnt?

(Guidance note: it is important for the hypnotherapist to validate and commend what the client has achieved as they remember what they have worked through)

I want to congratulate you on the progress you have made through your journey of grief. You have recognised what happened when you experienced *(the loss)*. With the strength that is deeply embedded within you, you have come to acknowledge the consequences for you and the effects it has had not only on your life – but also very importantly on your wellbeing. At times you may have felt disbelief – anger – lost – despondent *(insert any other emotion relevant to the client)* – but you came to believe that you would survive the journey. You have survived the journey. You are ready now to accept that things have changed and life cannot go back to how it was before *(the loss)*. You have taken so many steps to acceptance already. Is there anything else you need to do to fully accept what has happened?

(Guidance note: at this stage of the treatment plan it is likely that the client is at the acceptance stage and no more work needs to be done – apart from planning for the future. Therefore, it is very likely that the client will answer 'no' to the question. However, if they do need to do anything the hypnotherapist should work with this before using the final part of the script)

I want to congratulate you again for the progress you have made. You have accepted what has happened to you because of the loss you have experienced. Be proud of yourself – you have worked through your grief and faced many difficult things. Acknowledge the strength which is deeply embedded within you and use it to your benefit for the future. Now is the time to focus on the future – to think about your hopes and aspirations.

(Guidance note: the hypnotherapist can continue to work on specific aspirations using the questions which follow or this can be done in a separate session)

1 What are your hopes/aspirations for the future?
2 What do you want to achieve?
3 What do you want to do?
4 What do you want to see?
5 Who do you want to see?
6 Who would you like to meet?
7 Who would you like to have a conversation with?
8 What would you like to talk about?
9 Is there anything in particular you want to say or ask?
10 Where would you like to go?
11 Do you want to do this with anybody?
12 When would you like to do this?
13 Does it matter when you do this?
14 What do you need in your life to make you happy?

Appendix 31.1: Aspirations – questions, list and plan

Below is a series of questions the hypnotherapist can use to focus the client on their hopes and aspirations for the future. The hypnotherapist will undoubtedly take notes during the session, which can then be transcribed to make:

a)   A simple list of the aspirations
b)   A more detailed aspirations plan, which should be written up after the session and then give to the client to keep.

SECTION A: QUESTIONS

1   What are your hopes/aspirations for the future?

2   What do you want to achieve?

3   What do you want to do?

4   What do you want to see?

5   Who do you want to see?

6   Who would you like to meet?

7   Who would you like to have a conversation with?

8   What would you like to talk about?

9   Is there anything in particular you want to say or ask?

10   Where would you like to go?

11   Do you want to do this with anybody?

12 When would you like to do this?

13 Does it matter when you do this?

14 What do you need in your life to make you happy?

SECTION B: ASPIRATIONS LIST

ASPIRATIONS LIST

1.

2.

3.

4.

5.

6.

7.

8.

9.

10.

SECTION C: ASPIRATIONS PLAN

ASPIRATIONS PLAN

(To be given to the client)
Name of client:
Date developed:
Name of aspiration Any specific details Any time limit

1.

2.

3.

4.

5.

6.

7.

8.

9.

10.

Signature of client:
Date:
Time:

32 Preparing for the future

Introduction

The two scripts in this chapter should be used when a treatment plan is nearing the end and the therapy is almost complete. The client has worked through the loss, is accepting of it and ready to look to the future. The scripts enable the client to look and plan for the future and can be used in conjunction with the aspirations questions presented in the previous chapter. The first script also enables the client to check whether there are still things they need to deal with or get rid of and this can be done using the bumper cars before driving around the future.

The second script uses bungee jumping to leap into the future, but should not be used for anyone who has a fear of heights.

Script 1: Bumper cars

When you have been going through a difficult time there comes a point when you need to clear the way in order to move forward into the future. To do this sometimes you need to move things out of the way so that you can drive forward. I want you to imagine that you are spending the day at a fairground. This fairground has all the usual stalls, rides, food and drink. I want you to saunter around and enjoy the atmosphere – look at all the different things. Maybe you can see a carousel – a big wheel – a man on stilts – a coconut shy – the candy floss stall. As you enjoy sauntering along – not rushing just taking your time – I want you to be looking for the bumper car ride. Take your time – tell me when you see the bumper cars. Look for the rods sticking up from the back of each bumper car.

Go towards the bumper car ride and have a look at the different cars. Decide which one you would like to drive and then climb in. Get yourself settled – comfortable. Look around the inside of the bumper car – see the steering wheel and find the throttle. The throttle will manage the speed at which the bumper car will travel. You will be in control of the steering wheel and the throttle. You can choose how fast or slow you travel – how fast or slow you deal with things. Feel the steering wheel – become

DOI: 10.4324/9781032245706-36

familiar with it. Now feel the throttle. Remember you are in control. You can travel at whatever speed you want. You are going to drive and steer the bumper car – you will be in complete control. Now before you start, think about the things that have been hindering you or holding you back since you lost *(insert loss)*. You have done so well to deal with those things. It is now time to look to the future, but before you do that I just want you to check that there is nothing else you need to deal with. I wonder if there is anything at all – thoughts – feelings – people – situations – which you need to bump out of your life. Just think about that and I shall be quiet for a short while.

(Guidance note: the hypnotherapist should leave sufficient time for the client to reflect before proceeding further)

Now look at the other bumper cars. In the seats of some of the bumper cars you may see what you need to get rid of from your life – you are going to bump them out of your life. This is going to be fun. How many bumper cars do you need to bump?

(Guidance note: there may only be one as the client is nearing the end of the treatment plan)

So get ready now – decide which bumper car you are going to bump first. Tell me who or what is in the bumper car you have chosen. Right – ready – steady – go. Drive your bumper car towards the bumper car you have chosen – bump it and bump it again – move it out of the way. Keep bumping it until it is completely out of your way and you can no longer see it. How good does that feel? Bump – bump – bump. Tell me when you have finished bumping that car and when it is completely out of the way – and out of sight completely.

(Guidance note: the hypnotherapist repeats the bumping process if there are more cars that need to be dealt with)

Well done. You have bumped everything out of the way. You can now drive around – go in whichever direction you want – and no one is going to bump you. You are free to go in whichever direction you want – there is no-one or nothing that can hinder you or block your way. Start your journey into the future in the bumper car – go in whichever direction you want. Enjoy the ride. Go at whatever speed you like – fast or slow – it does not matter – it is your choice how you travel – you are in control of your future.

Script 2: Bungee jumping into the future

Today is the day to jump into your future. To feel free and exhilarated – looking forward to the future. You are going to bungee jump into your future. Looking to the future can be scary – just like bungee jumping might be a bit scary if you have not done it before. But doing something new – different – can also be very exciting.

Imagine that you are looking at a huge crane which has been positioned at the side of a very wide and deep lake. You see some people gathered at the bottom of the crane. You can also see what looks like a large steel box. Walk towards the crane. A man comes to greet you. You then walk with him towards the steel box, which you now realise is the lift that is going to take you up to the platform at the top of the crane. The man is going to help you get ready for your jump. He helps you put on a helmet, harness and ties the cords to your feet. He makes sure you are going to be very safe. For a moment you might feel a bit hesitant, but if that happens, you know it is only for a second or so. You know you want to jump into your future. There is a small gate into the steel box – go through that now – the man follows you through the gate and then he shuts the gate. The steel box starts to lift off the ground – it is moving upwards. See what a beautiful view you have – as the box moves up and up – up and up. Slowly and steadily. The steel box is sturdy and safe. Up and up – up and up you go. Look at the lake – what can you see? The trees – people – what else can you see? You feel excited – enjoy the anticipation – you are about to jump into your future.

The steel box is nearly at the platform now. Take a few deep breaths to prepare yourself. This jump is going to help you take a leap into the future. The steel box has stopped moving now. Walk through the gate onto the platform. The man will help you get attached to the crane. He will make it very safe for you. So you are ready. Stand on the platform. Look out across the lake. Think about what you want in your future. Now when you bungee jump you will drop head first and you may bounce up and down a few times. This will give you the chance to see the future but also to change anything you are not happy with. Ready now. On the count of 3, you are going to bungee jump – *1, 2, and 3* – jump.

Down you go – soaring into the future. Look into the lake – look across the lake. What do you see? Down and down you go. Tell me what you see as you are jumping into your future. What do you want in your future? You are still soaring down into your future. What is happening? What are you seeing? How are you feeling?

The cords are nearly at their full length – fully stretched. You can see clearly into the lake and across the lake – seeing the future. You are at full stretch now and then suddenly you bounce back upwards. You saw the future clearly. Is there anything you need to change right now for the future? If so, do it now. Make any changes to make the future just as you want it to be.

Now bounce back down again – and you bounce back up again. Keep looking into the lake – and across the lake – see the future. Whilst you are bouncing up and down think about whether there is anything you need to be different in the future? Now make any changes you want in order to make the future just as you want it to be. Think about changes you might need to make in the way you respond to things – how you think – how you feel – how you behave. You know you are capable of making changes – you have the motivation – the determination – and the strength – to live your life the way you want. Keep bouncing up and down – keep looking – make any changes you want.

(Guidance note: the hypnotherapist should work with the client to change anything whilst they are bouncing up and down)

The cords have finished bouncing up and down now. You can just swing for a while. Just enjoy swinging around – looking to the future – feel the excitement – you are so near the future now.

33 The jigsaw puzzle

Introduction

After experiencing a loss a person can feel very mixed up and not know what to do to make him/herself feel any better. Thinking about the future can seem impossible when everything seems unclear, muddled and confusing. The script below embeds the idea that things can become clearer by taking time to look carefully at all the individual pieces, which need to be put together to get the complete picture. The word 'torn' is used within the script rather than 'broken' as I feel strongly it is not helpful to the client to think they are or have been broken and need to be fixed.

The script

Imagine that you are sitting at a table. A table which is big enough to have lots of things spread out on it when needed. Look in front of you and you will see a pile of what looks like little bits of cardboard. Look closer – you realise the little bits of cardboard are pieces of a jigsaw puzzle. Look hard at the pile of pieces. Is that how you have been feeling? Torn apart – in pieces – mixed up – not fitting together – not seeing the whole picture. When you experience a loss it is natural to feel any of these things. Your emotions can pile up – become a heap of torn bits.

Look closer at the pile of jigsaw pieces in front of you. There are lots of pieces. The thought of putting the jigsaw together might feel quite daunting. There are just so many pieces to sort out and understand what the final picture should look like. You see there is no box for the pieces – no picture to look at – but I am sure you can work it out. Start moving the pile of jigsaw pieces around. Spread them out. Pick up some pieces – feel the texture – what they are made of. Do some pieces feel harder than others? Are some pieces really worn down – thin – bent – faded? Are some pieces torn? Keep moving the pieces around – spread them out. Look at them. What colours can you see? What shapes? Does anything make any sense yet? Keep moving the pieces around. Be patient. You will start to see what is on the pieces. Keep moving the pieces around. Take your time –

DOI: 10.4324/9781032245706-37

there is no need to rush. Take your time to look at the pieces and what is on them.

It can take time to see things clearly – to get the final picture. You may have been feeling muddled – lost – unsure *(insert anything else the client has mentioned)*. Like the jigsaw puzzle you may have been feeling torn apart – in pieces – mixed up – not fitting together – not seeing the whole picture. The pieces can be put together again – a picture will emerge. You just need to give yourself time and be patient. Think about how you feel now and how you want to feel in the future.

Look at the pieces on the table in front of you. What have you done with them so far? Pick up a piece now – look at it – really stare at it – and tell me what you see.

(Guidance note: the hypnotherapist should encourage the client to explain in detail what they see and how it makes him/her feel. The client should not be rushed)

Now pick up another piece – look at it – really stare at it – and tell me what you see?

(Guidance note: the hypnotherapist should let the client work with several pieces. Some useful prompts follow)

What are you seeing?
What is it making you think about?
How are you feeling as you are holding/looking at this piece?
You are beginning to see things more clearly. Feel that sense of purpose growing inside of you. You know you can put this jigsaw together – that it will all make sense in the end. You will see the full picture. Just be patient – no need to rush. When you are ready, I want you to start sorting the rest of the pieces. Spread them out. Pick them up. Look at them. Sort them out. Take your time. I am going to be quiet for a short while.

(Guidance note: the hypnotherapist should leave the client to sort the pieces for a few minutes)

Tell me when you are ready to start putting the jigsaw together – when you are ready to make the picture. If any of the pieces need repairing because they are torn or worn, find some glue or Sellotape you can use. Make the pieces ready for their purpose – to make a complete picture.

OK – now you are ready to put the jigsaw together. You will know exactly which piece fits with another piece and where to place them. As you start to fit the pieces together – tell me what you are seeing and tell me how you are feeling.

(Guidance note: it is important for the hypnotherapist to encourage the client to speak about what they are building as the picture)

The picture is coming together – it is becoming clearer – much clearer. Carry on until the picture is completed – all the pieces have been put together. Now tell me what you see.

(Guidance note: the hypnotherapist works with the client on the future i.e. how to achieve what the client is seeing as their future)

34 Kaleidoscope

Introduction

This script can help a client who has repetitive negative responses with regard to how they think, feel and behave. S/he may have developed certain habits in the way they are handling a loss (or losses). Through the kaleidoscope the client is encouraged to see repeating patterns and to make changes which will make the future (final pattern/image) better. Watching the patterns embeds the idea of change, movement, shifting and enlightenment.

The script

You are holding a kaleidoscope in your hand. Look at it – the tube is in two parts. There is one part you can turn and twist around. Look at the end where there is a hole to look through. A kaleidoscope is so interesting and intriguing. It can show you many things and it can make things come together to make lots of different patterns – the patterns keep changing – you will see things in a completely different way.

The kaleidoscope is a bit like life really. Living life shows you many things – you can look at those things from different angles – you can interpret things in a variety of ways – how you see them – and you can change the way you see them. The kaleidoscope uses light and mirrors to reflect objects and it can create both new and repeating patterns. You can repeat patterns – sometimes that is helpful and sometimes it is not. Repeating a pattern becomes unhelpful when you keep responding in a negative way and it becomes a habit. Sometimes you might make the same mistakes – but eventually you will learn from the mistakes. You need to change things by using the light – being enlightened by what you have learnt.

Lift the kaleidoscope up and hold it in front of you, so you can look through the hole in the end. Look into the kaleidoscope and tell me what you see. What colours – what shapes – what patterns. Now turn the tube and watch the colours – the shapes and patterns begin to change. Watch

DOI: 10.4324/9781032245706-38

the new patterns emerge. As you watch changes are taking place. You are becoming excited to see what happens next – what emerges – it is very exciting to see something new – new patterns forming. Keep turning the tube.

Take a rest for a minute from looking into the kaleidoscope. Think about what has been happening to you recently. What you have lost. How you have been feeling. Look into the kaleidoscope again and see what has been happening to you. Tell me what you see exactly.

(Guidance note: the hypnotherapist should let the client explain what they are seeing and then continue encouraging the client to turn the tube so that events which have occurred since the loss are seen and talked about. Usually there will be recurring patterns for the client – regarding their thought processes, how they have been feeling, how they have responded and behaved.

The hypnotherapist needs to work with the client to see these patterns)

Now turn the tube again and tell me what you see next. Tell me what you see exactly.

(Guidance note: keep repeating until all recent events associated with the loss have been seen and discussed fully)

You have been seeing patterns. You have seen how things have changed. Now it is time to change things for a better future. The loss you have experienced has already changed things for you. Now it is time to change things for you again – to make life better – just as you want to live it. So you are going to look into the kaleidoscope again and see the things you want in your life. You will keep turning the tube until the patterns and pictures you want to be in your future appear inside the kaleidoscope. Hold the kaleidoscope in front of you again and look through the hole. See the patterns changing. Watch the movement – watch the patterns – keep turning the tube – you will know when the patterns are just right for you. Use your enlightenment – think about what you have learnt over the past few weeks and months *(insert years if appropriate)*. Use the light – your enlightenment – to create new patterns – a new picture. Tell me what is happening. What do you see?

(Guidance note: the hypnotherapist then works with the client to see how they want their life to be in the future. There needs to be emphasis on enlightenment and creating new patterns of behaviour. Then the hypnotherapist should finish with some ego boosting)

35 Clouds coming together

Introduction

This script should be used when a client is coming towards the end of their journey of grief. The client will have accepted their loss and will have developed some understanding of how it has affected them. This script embeds the idea of merging experiences from the past and the present and then seeing the full picture, that is, the future.

The script

I want you to think about how things can fit together very naturally. Things come together for a reason. Imagine two beautiful pieces of wood that will dovetail together to make a piece of furniture, which is not only beautiful but also very solid. I wonder what is coming into your mind – what piece of furniture you are seeing. Think about other things that come together – fit together – and work well together. Like a plug fits into an electric socket and enables power and energy. Sometimes it takes time for things to come together – things may have to merge together gradually to become as one.

I want you to imagine you are lying on a bed in a room, which has a huge window. You are lying on your side looking out of the window. It is a lovely sunny day. From where you are lying – you see the vast sky through the window. Look at the blue sky through the window. I wonder what you see in the sky – birds flying so gracefully – up, down and around. Maybe aeroplanes or helicopters will be flying about too. There will be some white clouds in the sky somewhere. Just give them time to appear. One big white cloud will from the left and another big white cloud will come from the right. Just give the two big clouds time to appear. Tell me when they have come into your view.

OK – good. Now first look at the cloud on the left. Look at the shape of the cloud – look at the indentations around the edges. Look at the different shades of white within it – dark and light. Then look at the cloud on the right. Look at the shape of the cloud – look at the indentations

DOI: 10.4324/9781032245706-39

around the edges. Look at the different shades of white within it – dark and light.

Look deeper now into the cloud on the left. See everything that you have lost in the past *(weeks/months/years – insert time frame as appropriate)*. Put all those negative thoughts you have been having into the cloud. Put all the negative feelings you have been experiencing into that same cloud. There may be other things you want to put in the cloud too. Just take your time. I know this might be hard but stay with it – remember what you have been going through. Think about what you need to put in the cloud. Now tell me what you are putting in the cloud.

(Guidance note: the hypnotherapist works with the client to put thoughts, feelings and anything else in the cloud)

Turn your attention now to the cloud on the right. Visualise what you want to happen over the next few *(weeks/months/years as appropriate)*. You have been working so hard to deal with the loss(es) you have experienced. You know that things are getting better and will continue to get better as you accept the loss(es). Tell me what hopes you have for the future and put them in the cloud.

(Guidance note: the hypnotherapist should use this time to build on the work undertaken with the client in their treatment plan to date and encourage the client to talk more about their hopes for the future)

Now look at both big white clouds. You see that they are starting to move towards each other. Very, very slowly they are moving towards each other. Gently and slowly they are getting nearer to each other. Just watch how gently and slowly they move. Watch the edges – the indentations of each cloud. Getting closer and closer now – nearer and nearer – almost there. Watch now how the two clouds merge together so easily – they fit together – so smoothly – so effortlessly. Look at how the two clouds have merged together peacefully – without any effort at all. It was a natural thing for the two clouds to come together to form a huge, beautiful, white cloud.

And that is what you will do. You will bring the past and what you have lost to merge with the future, which is full of your hopes and aspirations. The past and the future can fit together to form something good – just like the two pieces of wood dovetail together to make a beautiful, solid piece of furniture. Or the plug and the electric socket that enable power and energy. Learn from the past – look to the future now – look at the beautiful enormous, fluffy white cloud that now exists.

36 Time capsule

Introduction

When something ends badly – like an important relationship – it is only natural for a person to focus on their most recent experiences; the experiences which maybe were unexpected and therefore hurtful or upsetting. At these times it can be hard to remember the good times. As time moves forward the emotional pain will ease and it will be possible to remember the good times and experiences. It is important to try to focus on the good times the person did experience and also to acknowledge what has been learnt from the experiences – good and bad. It is not healthy to dwell on the bad things because that habit of doing so can alter a person's perception; perhaps they become bitter, cynical or pessimistic. It is much healthier to focus on the good things and look back on and encapsulate the positives. Using the time capsule is a way of enabling this. The client remembers the positives about the person/relationship and is encouraged to talk about them before putting them in the time capsule, which stores the good memories and can be returned to at any time.

The script

You have been through a bad time with the loss of *(insert client's loss)* but I want you to remember the good things – the good times – the good experiences – and encapsulate them.

I want you to create a time capsule so you can put the good experiences and the lessons learnt into that capsule so they are a time in your life that you can look back on in a positive way. So on the count of *3*, I want you to see your time capsule – *1, 2,* and *3* – and there it is. Tell me what it looks like. The capsule is locked at the moment – can you see how it can be unlocked? On the count of *3*, I want you to unlock the capsule and look inside – *1, 2,* and *3*. Is anything inside the capsule already?

(Guidance note: if the client does find something in the capsule then the following exploratory questions should be used for each item)

DOI: 10.4324/9781032245706-40

Tell me what you have found.

What memory/experience does that bring back?

How do you feel when you think about the memory/experience?

Tell me more about what happened.

What is significant for you?

What did you learn from that experience?

What was good/positive about *(person/relationship/situation/experience)?*

What was bad/negative about *(person/relationship/situation/experience)?*

Do you want to keep *(what has been found)* in the time capsule?

If you do not want it in the time capsule, how are you going to dispose of it?

(Guidance note: if the client does want to dispose of an item, the hypnotherapist should ask how s/he wants to do this. The hypnotherapist then works with the client to do this before going on to the next item)

Now is the time to think about what you would like to put in the time capsule – what you want to keep. Think back to the good things that happened with *(insert as appropriate – person/relationship/situation).* Think about things you did.

(Guidance note: usually the client will remember some positives and the hypnotherapist should encourage them to talk in depth about each memory/ experience, which will then be encapsulated within the time capsule. Below is a list of ideas which can be used as prompts if required)

- Significant events e.g. personal, social or work
- Gigs, theatre, cinema, museum, restaurants, shops
- Incidents
- Conversations
- Trips/visits/holidays.

Now think about what you want to put in the time capsule to help you remember each good memory that you have been talking about. What would you like to put in the capsule?

(Guidance note: usually the client will identify things to go in the time capsule. Below are some typical examples, which can be used as prompts if required)

- Ticket
- Programme
- Cutting from a newspaper
- Item of clothing
- Hair
- Toy/doll
- Jewellery
- Possession/item

- Photograph
- Letter/note/card
- Poem
- Recording: audio or visual.

Are you absolutely sure that you have put everything you want in the time capsule? Just take a moment and think again about the good memories. Are you ready now to close the time capsule? OK – now close the time capsule. Lock or seal it *(depending on what the client has identified as the time capsule)*. Only you can open the time capsule because everything in it belongs to you – it is full of your good memories. Any time you want to remember just come back to the time capsule and open it. Now where would you like to put the time capsule for safe keeping?

(Guidance note: the hypnotherapist works with the client to put the time capsule in a safe place where it can be returned to in the future)

37 Brightness on the horizon

Introduction

Clients may seek the help of a hypnotherapist as a last resort when they are feeling utter despair. It is quite common for a client to have previously visited various counsellors and therapists before seeking the help and expertise of a hypnotherapist. The job of any hypnotherapist is to promote positivity and work towards creating goals based on the hopes and aspirations of the client. When a client is in despair s/he may feel that everything is pointless, that is, there is no hope for the future. The script below was written to give hope and encourage optimism.

The script

You are sitting somewhere where you are looking out to the horizon. It does not matter where you are exactly – you are feeling calm as you look towards the horizon where the bottom of the sky meets the land or perhaps it meets the sea. I do not know but you know that this is your horizon and you know what it looks like. So keep looking at your horizon – the more you look at it, the calmer you feel.

I know you have not been feeling very good recently. You have been feeling very low *(insert any other feelings the client has discussed – use their exact words if possible)* and as though there is little to look forward to in the future. Feeling like that can make you tired and lethargic – it is an effort to do anything – but I know you want things to change and be better. I know that for sure, otherwise you would not be sitting here – feeling calm – and looking out to your horizon. Keep looking at your horizon.

Look at the bottom of the sky – concentrate – focus. You start to see something yellow pop up – a bit of bright yellow. It rises up a little bit more. As you see the yellow rise up into your horizon you feel lighter. Yellow is such a bright colour – it is cheerful – it makes you feel good. Keep watching the yellow – the brightness – rising up and up. As it rises more and more you realise that it is the sun that is rising up – it is

DOI: 10.4324/9781032245706-41

dawning. The sun rises at the beginning of every single day. It is reliable – the light will always follow the dark. Lightness will always follow the darkness. Watch the sun rise further – higher and higher it goes – reaching for the sky. As it goes higher, focus on the brightness. You start to feel hopeful – optimistic – you feel a brightness rising within you. That brightness which is expanding within you is excluding all the darkness you have been feeling. Soon all the darkness will have disappeared completely and all that will be left within you will be brightness.

So now that you are feeling hopeful and optimistic. Think about the future. Think about things you would like to do – things you want to achieve. Take your time and think about those things now. Think about your future with hope and optimism – knowing you can achieve anything because you have that brightness inside of you – shining continuously.

(Guidance note: the hypnotherapist should then work with the client to define exactly what they want for their future)

What do you want to do in the future?
What do you want to achieve?
Where do you want to go?
How do you want to feel?
How soon do you want this to happen?
How will you make it happen?
What changes do you need to make?

Continue to sit and watch the brightness on the horizon – your horizon. You can come and sit here at any time and enjoy the brightness – feel hopeful – feel optimistic – and look forward to the future.

(Guidance note: it can be beneficial to finish the session with some ego boosting)

Part V
Additional scripts

38 Being assertive

Introduction

One of the most common problems presented to a hypnotherapist is the loss of confidence or someone saying they have never been a confident person and their self-esteem is really low. Experiencing any loss can result in a person feeling less confident, unsure what to do and questioning themselves. It is going to be even harder for someone who has never had any self-belief or confidence in themselves. A hypnotherapist can work on confidence using any number of techniques; such techniques can also be put to good use when helping a client with a loss. In addition, it can be beneficial to include a session on being more assertive. This is why I have included this chapter and a script about becoming assertive, which teaches some basic assertiveness skills.

It is important to work on building confidence and for a client to feel better about him/herself when dealing with any number of situations. However, when dealing with any loss it may become equally important for the client to develop some assertiveness skills and confront situations they might previously have avoided. How many times have you heard someone say: 'I hate confrontation'? Hypnotherapy can help a client to feel confident about dealing with or confronting a person or situation, but s/he needs the tools to do it. The importance of the language used (i.e. words and phrases) and body language needs to be taught and understood in order to become more assertive. Ideally going on a one-day face-to-face assertiveness training course is the best way to learn and practise techniques, but certain things can be learnt and rehearsed whilst in the trance state. I do run assertiveness courses and over the years have written scripts for individual hypnotherapy sessions. I think it is helpful for some work to be done on building confidence before using the script below in a separate session.

When I work on assertiveness with a hypnotherapy client, I do some of the preparatory work in the conscious state. For example, it is very important to talk about 'rights', so I usually give the client a handout[1] (see Appendix 38.1) and these rights are revisited when in trance. The client

DOI: 10.4324/9781032245706-43

then develops their own 'personal' rights whilst in trance. I have included a form as Appendix 38.2, which can be used by the hypnotherapist to list the original rights, any further rights developed and mantras created during the hypnotherapy session. The hypnotherapist can use the form during a session to make notes. It can then be typed up properly afterwards and a copy given to the client to keep.

It can be useful to make a recording of the script after the session has taken place (making it directly relevant and individual to the client) so the client can use it for practise before the next session.

The script

I want to congratulate you on how you have been building your confidence and the progress you have been making. You have been working and practising really hard and I know you have made changes *(insert some examples if possible)*. I am seeing such a change in you as a whole. Another thing I think we should give some attention to is the subject of assertiveness and how you can become more assertive. Many people recoil at that word – assertiveness. Often this is because they confuse it with the word aggression. Being assertive is not about being aggressive, so I want us to concentrate on this today and learn some simple techniques and develop some mantras.

Relax your body – which maybe has gone a little tense since I mentioned the word assertiveness. You know don't you that when you relax your body – your mind relaxes too? The more you relax the more your subconscious mind relaxes and becomes more receptive to accept suggestions to improve your wellbeing. Keep breathing in and out slowly as you know how to do so well now.

I want you to think about what you have achieved in your hypnotherapy sessions – how confident you have become – and commend yourself. Now you need to take another step forward and work towards becoming more assertive. Everybody has the right to express themselves and ask for what they want. Do you remember how we discussed your rights? As you keep relaxing there – going deeper and deeper into trance – I am going to repeat those rights to you and while I do that, I want you think about what they mean to you. I want you to remember that you have the right:

- To set your own objectives and priorities
- To state your own needs
- To ask for what you want
- To express your feelings
- To voice your opinions and values
- To say 'yes' or 'no' for yourself
- To make mistakes
- To change your mind

- To say when you don't understand
- To decline responsibility for other people's problems
- To be listened to
- To be treated with respect
- To put yourself first if you need to do so
- To stand up for and fight for your rights
- To feel good about yourself.

I am going to repeat each one of these rights again – one by one. After each one, I want you tell me what you are thinking about in relation to that particular right – what you are good at or what you need to work on or improve upon.

(Guidance note: the hypnotherapist should have Appendix 38.2 to hand so s/he can repeat each right and have discussion in between each one. The appendix can be used to take notes. Some questions are listed below for use if needed)

What are you thinking about this particular right?
What are you good at in relation to this right?
Do you think you need to work on any aspect of this right?
What do you need to work on?
What could be improved upon?
How are you going to do this?
What do you need to do?
What do you need to stop doing?

(Guidance note: once all the rights have been revisited, the script continues enabling the hypnotherapist to ask the client if s/he wants to add any more personalised rights to the original list. Again Appendix 38.2 can be used to take notes)

Is there anything you would like to add to the list of rights? Anything that is important or particularly relevant to you – your situation. Just think about that for a while. Think about rights which are personal to you – your own personal rights.

(Guidance note: the hypnotherapist should repeat any additions in the session and write them up in full after the session has finished using a fresh copy of Appendix 38.2)

OK so you know what you need to work on over the next few days and weeks regarding your rights and I want you to say a mantra frequently to yourself or out loud: I have rights. Say that out loud now: I have rights. And again: I have rights. Say your mantra with confidence – feel the confidence inside of you. Say it – believe it: I have rights.

Just keep relaxing but at the same time start to feel that you are becoming more assertive. To be assertive you need to think about the language you use – words and phrases – and how you say things. To do this you need to: think – prepare – rehearse. That is another good mantra to say to yourself or out loud: think – prepare – rehearse. Say that out loud now: think – prepare – rehearse. As you say your mantras, imagine yourself saying them assertively and imagine how you are looking when you are being assertive. You need to make yourself clear – be direct – do not waffle – do not get side-tracked – do not be derailed by anyone. So just think about that a little more deeply. You need to make yourself clear – be direct – do not waffle – do not get side-tracked – do not be derailed by anyone.

You need to think about what you want to say – how you will say it – and then say it slowly – there is no need to rush through your sentences. Slow down the way you speak. Space out your words. It can help to have a structure for what you want to say, so you do not lead up to things or go all around the houses – waffle – or pad things out.

There are three things you need to do to have a simple structure:

- Acknowledge what the person has said or done
- Explain how it (their words or actions) made you feel
- Say what you want them to do or what you want them to change (e.g. their behaviour).

You need to keep this simple. Keep your sentences short and to the point. The three things you need to do are:

- Acknowledge what the person has said or done
- Explain how it (their words or actions) made you feel
- Say what you want them to do or what you want them to change (e.g. their behaviour).

Keep your sentences short and to the point – remember no waffle or padding out. As you are thinking about each of these things you are becoming more assertive – more and more assertive. Feel that assertiveness growing inside you. There will be things you need to stop doing too in order to become more assertiveness. I wonder if:

- You have ever counted how many times you say 'sorry'
- You apologise when you have nothing to apologise for
- You repeat yourself
- You feel you have to justify yourself
- You make excuses.

Remember – you will not:

- Apologise – say sorry
- Lead up to what you want to say – go all around the houses

- Waffle
- Pad out
- Repeat yourself
- Get distracted
- Get derailed by someone
- Feel you have to justify yourself
- Make excuses.

Remember the structure – just three things:

- Acknowledge what the person has said or done
- Explain how it (their words or actions) made you feel
- Say what you want them to do or what you want them to change (e.g. their behaviour).

As you are thinking about these things you are becoming more assertive – more and more assertive. Feel that assertiveness growing inside you. Now think back to recent events since you experienced *(the loss)*. Think about a situation you found yourself in. Reflect on what happened – what you did – what you said. Think about how you could have dealt with the situation better or expressed yourself more assertively. Now tell me what happened exactly.

(Guidance note: the hypnotherapist should encourage the client to give as much detail as possible about what was said [exploring the words used]; and what was done)

Now think about what you would say or do differently. Think about the three things you need to do and imagine what you would say and how you would look as you speak:

- Acknowledge what the person has said or done
- Explain how it (their words or actions) made you feel
- Say what you want them to do or what you want them to change (e.g. their behaviour).

To become more assertive it can be good to: think – prepare – rehearse. This could be another mantra for you to use: think – prepare – rehearse. Say that now out loud: think – prepare – rehearse. And again: think – prepare – rehearse.

(Guidance note: the hypnotherapist then goes through each stage and gets the client to think, prepare and rehearse what they are going to say. It is essential that the hypnotherapist gives feedback – especially if some wordage used is not assertive)

Good – that sounds great. Now imagine how you look when you are saying what you need to say.

How are you positioned – standing or sitting?
What expression have you got on your face?
Are you looking directly into the person's eyes?
Are you maintaining eye contact?
How long do you maintain eye contact for?
Watch your breathing – are you breathing calmly and gently?
Do you need to slow down your breathing?

Now I want you to practise another mantra: I am assertive – I am not aggressive. Say that now out loud: I am assertive – I am not aggressive. And again: I am assertive – I am not aggressive. Good. Now is there a mantra you would like to create yourself and use?

(Guidance note: if the client does create another mantra or more mantras in future sessions they should be added to Appendix 38.2)

Well done. You have thought about a lot of things today and from this day forward you are going to become more and more assertive. As this happens you are going to think – prepare – rehearse – so that day by day it becomes so easy for you to be assertive. Eventually you will not think about it at all – being assertive will come so naturally to you.

Note

1 Developed from the original work of Anne Dickson (1982) *A Woman in Your Own Right: Assertiveness and You.* London: Quartet Books. Updated Anniversary version printed 2012.

Appendix 38.1: Handout – I have rights

I HAVE RIGHTS

- To set my own objectives and priorities
- To state my own needs
- To ask for what I want
- To express my feelings
- To voice my opinions and values
- To say 'yes' or 'no' for myself
- To make mistakes
- To change my mind
- To say when I don't understand
- To decline responsibility for other people's problems
- To be listened to
- To be treated with respect
- To put myself first if I need to do so
- To stand up for and fight for my rights
- To feel good about myself.

Appendix 38.2: Form for rights and mantras

RIGHTS

- To set my own objectives and priorities
- To state my own needs
- To ask for what I want
- To express my feelings
- To voice my opinions and values
- To say 'yes' or 'no' for myself
- To make mistakes
- To change my mind
- To say when I don't understand
- To decline responsibility for other people's problems
- To be listened to
- To be treated with respect
- To put myself first if I need to do so
- To stand up for and fight for my rights
- To feel good about myself.

Additional rights created during a hypnotherapy session

1.

2.

3.

4.

5.

6.

7.

8.

9.

10.

Mantras

1.

2.

3.

4.

5.

Name of client:
Date:

39 Freedom

Perhaps many of us take for granted the freedom we have to live our lives as we wish to do. Maybe that is a human failing for many of us and the saying: 'You never know what you've got until it is missing' rings very true. In many societies across the world people are fortunate to live their lives freely, but sadly there are still societies that place massive restrictions on their citizens. I think it is helpful to remind ourselves that in our society we are fortunate to have the *Human Rights 1998*[1] and to remember Article 2 promotes the right to life:

1 Everyone's right to life shall be protected by law. No one shall be deprived of his life intentionally save in the execution of a sentence of a court following his conviction of a crime for which this penalty is provided by law.
2 Deprivation of life shall not be regarded as inflicted in contravention of this Article when it results from the use of force which is no more than absolutely necessary:
    (a) in defence of any person from unlawful violence;
    (b) in order to effect a lawful arrest or to prevent the escape of a person lawfully detained;
    (c) in action lawfully taken for the purpose of quelling a riot or insurrection.

I also think it is helpful to remember and use famous quotes from people who have experienced losing their rights or freedom. I encourage many of my clients to develop their own affirmations and mantras, but in some hypnotherapy sessions I do incorporate meaningful quotes. Some examples being:

> There is no easy walk to freedom anywhere, and many of us will have to pass through the valley of the shadow of death again and again before we reach the mountain top of our desires.
>
> Nelson Mandela (1995)[2]

DOI: 10.4324/9781032245706-44

If you can't fly then run, if you can't run then walk, if you can't walk then crawl, but whatever you do you have to keep moving forward.

Martin Luther King (1960)[3]

This chapter will firstly consider the different ways freedom can be lost from childhood through to later adulthood and where this might happen, the objective being that the hypnotherapist can be more prepared to work with some of these situations. Freedom will mean different things to people in a variety of situations, so when working with a client it is important to ascertain what freedom means to them. It begs some crucial questions:

What have you lost?
What happened to you?
How has this affected you?
What does freedom mean to you?
In what way(s) do you want to be free in the future?

If working with a group it can be useful to get clients to verbalise or write down what freedom means to them and after discussion give them a handout with a list of definitions. This work is done in the conscious state, before using hypnosis. Some dictionary definitions of freedom are:

- the power or right to act, speak, or think as one wants
- the state of not being imprisoned or enslaved

(Oxford English Dictionary)[4]

- the condition or right of being able or allowed to do, say, think, etc. whatever you want to, without being controlled or limited

(Cambridge English Dictionary)[5]

- the state of being free or at liberty rather than in confinement or under physical restraint
- exemption from external control, interference, regulation, etc.
- the power to determine action without restraint
- political or national independence
- personal liberty, as opposed to bondage or slavery
- exemption from the presence of anything specified.

(www.dictionary.com)[6]

Examples of presenting situations

A hypnotherapist could have to work with losses which have been experienced by a client recently or a very long time ago. Having restrictions placed on one's freedom is a loss; some examples of such situations which might need to be worked on are:

- Strict or overprotective parents: not allowing a child to play out or to socialise with peers/friends; setting time restrictions/curfew
- Controlling partner/family/relatives: due to tradition/cultural expectations
- School: not being able to attend a school of choice; not being able to study certain subjects
- Manager who bullies a worker and restricts opportunities for learning experiences, developing knowledge/skills or promotion
- Perpetrator of abuse using power and control:

  - Domestic abuse: coercion and control
  - Modern slavery: gangmaster/lieutenant locking workers in accommodation; transported to and from workplace
  - Forced marriage: potential victim is being followed/escorted everywhere; locked in a room until the ceremony takes place

- Having no options to change/do things because of deficits e.g. money; disability
- Imprisoned during war/holocaust
- Covid-19 pandemic: lockdown/restrictions.

Places/institutions where it feels like freedom has been lost

When thinking of places where freedom could be denied it is very easy to immediately think of institutions, but movement could be restricted in so many places. People who have lost their freedom physically can talk about having their minds, thinking and speech restricted. Freedom could be lost in:

- Own home: locked in a cupboard; confined to one room; not allowed to have choice about food to be eaten, television programmes to watch.
- A place where a person is forced to sleep
- Children's home/residential unit
- Young offenders unit/secure unit/prison
- Hospital
- Psychiatric facility
- Addiction rehabilitation centre
- Residential/nursing home.

There are a lot of clients who may feel they have lost their freedom or they have been incarcerated in the past and feel very cheated. They may feel they have lost time, a part of their life or opportunity. They could feel a lot of different emotions (e.g. bitter; angry; resentful; jealous) and have regrets. It can be a vital part of a treatment plan to explore these emotions and create some hope and goals for the future. I think a hypnotherapist can offer a vital service to people who feel there is no hope for the future as everything has been lost or ended.

A person can feel they have lost their freedom (i.e. the choice to live their life how they would wish to do) through no fault of their own. A classic example would be a child who was taken into care because their parents could not look after them. The child has then be placed in a children's home or moved frequently around different foster parents. This can result in loss of stability and loss of faith in the system/workers. Older people may have lived through so many life experiences where they lost their freedom:

- Having tuberculosis/polio as a child and being isolated in a hospital for a very long time
- War: prisoner of war; citizen not living their life freely because of civil unrest or war
- Being in hospital later in life: due to stroke, heart attack or ongoing illness
- Being placed in a care/nursing home.

The hypnotherapist will usually develop a treatment plan after an initial assessment. Some common objectives which may be written into such a plan might be to achieve freedom from:

- Fear
- Harm
- Restraint
- Any limitations.

What follows is a mixture of longer and shorter scripts; all of which aim to encourage the client to think about what freedom means to him/her and how to achieve it. There is a general introduction to trance, which can be used with the three main scripts. Script 2 focuses more on release of thoughts, feelings or behaviours. Script 3 again focuses on achieving freedom. The short additional script works on fortitude can be used as a follow on from Script 3. Finally, a short visualisation is included which addresses the feeling of being trapped and then escaping.

General introduction to trance

Make yourself comfortable. Close your eyes when you are ready. Slow your breathing down – that's right. Breathe very slowly. Just take a gentle breath in – don't gulp – and then gently breathe out – that's right. Breathe in and breathe out. Good. Feel your body starting to relax. Keep breathing slowing – slow your breathing right down. Breathe in and breathe out.

Even when you feel physically trapped and incapacitated, you can always escape in your mind. Your clever subconscious mind can take you anywhere you want to go. There are no limits – no walls to keep you in. By going into trance you can take yourself away from the conscious state and enjoy travelling in your imagination.

Script 1: The compass

Just squeeze your eyelids very tight and then gently relax them. Yes that's right. Do that again. Squeeze your eyelids very very tight and then gently relax them. One more time. Squeeze your eyelids very very tight and then gently relax them. Now on the count of *3*, I want you to imagine that you are opening your eyes. Feel that excitement rising within you – knowing you are going to see something new and be able to go in a different direction. Ready now – *1, 2,* and *3*. Imagine that you are opening your eyes and then look down – you are standing on something very big and round. You know you are standing on a big circle. Keep looking at the circle – look at the floor – see what it is made of – look at what colour or colours you can see on the floor of the circle.

You keep looking at the floor. You feel a sense of lightness around you. You also feel that sense of excitement again. Start to walk around the circle. You see four big letters written on the circle – equally spaced out. You will see – N – E – S – and W. Walk right around the circle – it does not matter which way you go. Just look deep into each letter as you go. Keep walking around the circle. Do that as many times as you like. You are free to do so. Keep walking around the circle. Enjoy the freedom.

Now look at the centre of the circle. You will see a huge pointer. You realise you are standing on a compass. A compass will point you in the right direction. You know you are safe when you have a compass because you know in which direction you are going. Now I know you have been feeling like you have lost direction recently. You are unsure which way to go. You have this compass to help you decide which direction you want to take. So look at the pointer. Ask it to point you in the right direction – the direction which is right for you. Watch the pointer – it will start to move. There is no need for it to rush. It may move around – change direction for a while – or change direction as many times as it needs to do – to the right – the left – clockwise – anti-clockwise. I do not know exactly – you just need to keep watching the pointer. What I do know is that it will eventually point you in the right direction. So, just keep watching the pointer and tell me when it has stopped moving and it is pointing in one direction.

OK – so look in the direction the pointer is pointing – and start walking in that direction. As you are walking you are feeling excited because you know you are moving forward – finding a new direction – a new purpose. You are feeling very excited – something you may not have felt for a while. At the same time you are feeling optimistic – confident in the knowledge that things are going to be better for you. Keep walking forward – feeling excited – optimistic and confident. Now keep walking and look for the future. You will see in front of you the right direction to take – your future. On the count of *3* everything will become very clear – you will know what you need to do – which direction to take. Now – *1, 2,* and *3*. What do you see?

> *(Guidance note: the hypnotherapist will then work with the client using what they are seeing/sensing as the right direction to take. The hypnotherapist can help the client to set goals for the future. It is helpful to anchor the compass for use in the future when the client needs to make a decision regarding which way to go – regarding any aspect of their life)*

Script 2: Releasing chains and padlocks

Today you are going to appear on a talent show. You are going to amaze the audience with just how easy you find it to get rid of things that are restricting you.

You are standing in the wings of a theatre. You see the stage in front of you. You stick your head around the big curtain and have a look at the audience. You can see lots of people – men, women, boys and girls – eagerly awaiting the next performance. Become aware of how you feel standing in the wings. You have lots and lots of chains wrapped around different parts of your body – your neck – the trunk of your body – each individual arm but your hands are free – each individual leg but your feet are free. Feel the weight of the chains – weighing down the whole of your body. The chains are like *(insert whatever is appropriate)* which have been tying you down – holding you back – making you feel as though you cannot go forward *(insert any other feelings which have been discussed)*. Chains feel like bonds that can never be broken. The many chains around your body are made of different metals – some thick some thin – and they are of different lengths – their links are different shapes and sizes. All the chains around your body are locked by padlocks.

It is nearly time for your performance to begin. I know this is going to be very hard to do but you need to walk towards the centre of the stage. You can see in the centre of the stage there is a table with a glass jar on it. Walking is going to be hard to do because the chains are so heavy – it feels like they weigh a ton – making it so difficult to walk. Start to walk now – drag your feet and body to the centre of the stage. I know it is hard – you feel weighed down by the chains but you can do this. Walk to the centre of the stage. You have the strength and determination to do this – no matter how hard it feels – how impossible it feels. Go on – keep going – drag your feet and body to the centre of the stage. Now you are there – well done.

Look at the expectant audience and smile at them. You are going to amaze them with your performance. Look at the glass jar on the top of the table. It is full of keys – keys for the padlocks which are keeping the chains wrapped around your body. Take a deep breath and look at each individual padlock around your body. Take your time – look at each padlock one at a time. Each padlock and the chain it is holding around your body represents something, someone or a situation *(or insert something in particular which has been discussed/is an issue)* that has made you feel weighed down – restricted. Now is the time to free yourself. Start the performance.

Take your time. Look at a padlock. See which chain it is keeping locked – a chain that has kept you restricted in your life. See what the chain is – something, someone or a situation – see the chain for what it is. Now reach into the glass jar and find the key to unlock the padlock. You know instinctively which is the right key to unlock the padlock. When you have found the key unlock that particular padlock. As it pops open the chain falls from your body onto the floor. Feel some of the heaviness fall away from you. The audience cheers.

Now look at another padlock. See which chain it is keeping locked – a chain that has kept you restricted in your life. See what the chain is – something, someone or a situation – see the chain for what it is. Now reach into the glass jar and find the key to unlock that padlock. You know instinctively which is the right key to unlock the padlock. When you have found the key unlock that particular padlock. As it pops open the chain you have been looking at drops down but this time even more chains fall from your body onto the floor. Feel some of the heaviness fall away from you. The audience cheers again. They are amazed that you know exactly which key fits which padlock. You know exactly what to do. There is no hesitation at all. You know how to unlock the padlocks. So keep doing that.

See each padlock – see the chains that have been restricting you. Remember how you have been feeling. How you have been chained up in your mind. Now is the time to get rid of all those chains that have been weighing you down and all the padlocks that have kept you locked in. Keep performing for the audience. Hear their excitement and cheers – urging you on and on – setting yourself free without any hesitation. Knowing exactly what must be done to become chain-free. Feel all the weights and heaviness lifting from you as the chains fall to the floor. Keep going – the chains and padlocks keep falling to the floor. Keep going until you are completely free of every single chain and padlock. Look at how excited the audience is getting – encouraging you – cheering you on. You are nearly completely free now – just a few more chains to get rid of. The last padlock and chains fall away. The audience goes mad – they stand on their feet shouting and clapping. You start swinging your arms about. You walk around the stage. You are completely free – nothing is restricting you or holding you back. Keep swinging your arms as you start running round the stage – completely free. Look at the audience – you have a standing ovation.

Script 3: Freedom on the mountainside

I am sure you have probably seen at some time – either on the television or in a film or in a photo in a magazine – that huge sign on top of a mountain that says 'Hollywood'. Even if you have not seen this landmark I want you to imagine it now. The word 'Hollywood' spelt out big and tall on top of a mountainside. It is an important sign – it welcomes people to Hollywood and lets them know they have arrived.

Look at that word now. Then you are going to change it so it becomes your landmark – your very own landmark. On the count of *3*, you will change the word 'Hollywood'. *1, 2,* and *3* – change the word to 'freedom'. See the word 'freedom'. Big and tall. Your word – your landmark.

So look at the word 'freedom' on top of the mountainside. Look at each letter very slowly – one by one: F – R – E – E – D – O – M. Think about what freedom means to you.

What do you need in your life to make you feel completely free?
What do you need to do to feel completely free?
What do you need to say (and to whom) to feel completely free?

Look at each letter very slowly again: F – R – E – E – D – O – M. It's time to make your way to freedom. Think about the things you need in your life – the things you need to do – the things you need say. You want to be free – you want to feel free – you want to experience freedom. Start now – make your way towards the bottom of the mountain and then start climbing up the mountainside. As you go higher and higher you feel freer and freer. Free to do whatever you like – live your life as you wish to do. Keep climbing. Just before you reach the top I want you to stop and stand still. Tell me when you are almost there.

OK – stand very still now. The word freedom is towering above you – seven very tall letters: F – R – E – E – D – O – M. In a moment you are going to stand on the top of the mountainside – are you ready? *1, 2,* and *3* – climb onto the top of the mountainside. The word freedom vanishes and you see your freedom. You are totally free.

(Guidance note: the hypnotherapist then works with what the client is seeing. The following questions can be used if required)

What are you seeing?
What does freedom look like to you?
How are you feeling right now?
What are you feeling now that you are completely free?
What are you thinking now?
What has the climb up the mountainside made you think about?
What have you come to realise?
Is there anything you need to do to maintain this feeling of freedom for the future?
Do you need to speak with anyone?
What do you need to say?
Is there anything you need to let go of? *(e.g. memory, thought, feeling?)*

You can see your future clearly now. You are free to enjoy your future and the freedom that you now have.

(Guidance note: the hypnotherapist can choose to continue and use the following additional script in the same session. Alternatively, the mountainside can be returned to in a future session)

Additional script: Fortitude

Fortitude is such a good word. It is such a powerful word. It means courage and emotional strength in the face of any pain or adversity. You have been going through a lot of pain because of *(insert loss)*. You are working towards accepting the loss and getting on with living your life in a way which is best for you. You can do this. You know you can do this. You have the courage to do this. You have the fortitude.

I want you to focus on the word 'fortitude'. I want you to see it written on top of the mountainside. See the word as a whole – 'fortitude'. Now concentrate on one letter at a time.

F – O – R – T – I – T – U – D – E

As you look at the word 'fortitude' you feel courage building up inside of you. Look at each individual letter again – very slowly. As you do so, feel that courage building up inside of you.

F – O – R – T – I – T – U – D – E

Feel courage increasing inside of you.

Now I want you take your time and build on this courage. I want you to look at each individual letter again. Look at the shape of the letter and then think what the letter might stand for. Remember fortitude means courage and emotional strength in the face of pain or adversity. You are building up your courage and emotional strength. Each individual letter will suggest what you need to do.

F = fight
O = organise
R = rebel
T = try
I = incite
T = trust
U = understand
D = determination
E = engage.

Look at the letters again. I wonder if you can think of any other meanings for each letter to increase your courage and emotional strength.

Let's start with F. What does the letter suggest to you to increase your courage and emotional strength?

> *(Guidance note: the hypnotherapist will take the client through each letter again and encourage more suggestions to reinforce the idea of increasing courage and emotional strength)*

Additional visualisation: The caged bird

You see in front of you a birdcage hanging from the ceiling. I wonder what shape it is. I wonder what it is made of. One thing I do know is that there is a small door somewhere in the cage – and that door is shut tight. Look into the cage now – you will see a bird – sitting on a perch. The bird is sitting very still. Look how still the bird is. You can just see it breathing – very slowly. Look at its feathers moving – up and down. Look at the colour of the feathers as they move up and down. The bird looks so still – it looks very passive. The bird's eyes do not move. It does not seem natural. It is not natural to be trapped in a cage – unable to get out. A bird should be free – free to fly – high in the sky or to anywhere else it needs to go. A bird should be able to walk on the ground – swim in water – go wherever it wants – do whatever it wants. I wonder what the bird is thinking as it sits so still – trapped in the cage. I wonder how the bird feels being locked in the cage. I wonder what emotions are trapped in that bird.

It is time to set the bird free. Look at the door of the cage and open it. The bird turns around and looks at the open door. It just keeps looking at the open space. It does not move – it just keeps looking outwards. Then the bird starts to look around – maybe checking out if it is safe to leave the cage. The bird starts to breathe quicker – you can see its feathers moving. The bird is looking very uncertain – it keeps looking around and then at the open space where the door was shut. It starts breathing even quicker – and then suddenly it flies off the perch and into the space. It flies through the open cage door. It is out of the cage. It is free. It flies fast. It flies high. It has escaped. It is free.

Notes

1 Human Rights Act 1998, Article 2, https://www.legislation.gov.uk/ukpga/1998/42/schedule/1/part/I/chapter/1
2 Nelson Mandela (1995) *Long Walk To Freedom: The Autobiography of Nelson Mandela* London: Abacus
3 This quote was taken from a speech given at a rally at Spelman College in April 1960.
4 Oxford Compact English Dictionary (2008) Oxford: Oxford University Press
5 https://dictionary.cambridge.org/dictionary/english/freedom
6 https://www.dictionary.com/browse/freedom

40 Bank vault

Introduction

The main script gets the client into a trance state and is a deepener. It is for use with a client who has suffered a loss and as a result has a lot going on in their life which needs sorting out and is taking up a lot of their time. Consequently, the client has little time for him/herself. The script introduces the idea of getting away from it all (the busy-ness or the business – the hypnotherapist can choose how they want to use the concept and words) and having some time alone. The additional scripts can then be used to work on specific issues.

Additional script 1 is for clients who say they have so many things to deal with and no time for themselves. Very often when a loss has been experienced a person likes to keep busy and this results in them putting themselves under pressure. In different circumstances, other people can be putting pressure on the client, who then feels stressed. The script facilitates slowing down and prioritising in order to reduce the busy-ness.

Additional script 2 has been included for hypnotherapists who want to use regression to work with a client.

The script

You are standing outside a bank. I do not know where this bank is exactly but you will know – and that is all that matters. The bank has large doors – people are coming in and out. On the outside wall of the bank there is a cash machine and some people are queuing up to get some money out. You can do all sorts of things when you are in a bank – draw money out – deposit cash or cheques – maybe talk to somebody and get some good advice about the best way to save, get a loan or a mortgage. Banks also store things and today you are going to explore this bank's vault which is underneath the building. The vault of the bank holds money but it also stores people's possessions – it keeps them very secure and safe. I think it might be useful for you to visit the vault to see what you find there.

DOI: 10.4324/9781032245706-45

Go through the front doors of the bank. Have a look around. You will see a lot of people – customers – staff who work in the bank – some will be greeting customers as they enter the bank – others will be working behind the counters. There will be more cash machines inside the bank too. People are standing – others are sitting on comfortable sofas – waiting patiently. The bank feels very busy. You need to find the way to the vault. There will be a door somewhere which leads to a staircase. Look for the door – when you see it walk towards it and then go through it. You will find yourself standing at the top of a staircase. It is very peaceful at the top of the staircase – away from the busy-ness of the bank. There is lots of work to be done in a bank – lots of business. You have been very busy lately since you lost *(insert loss)*. Now is the time to have some time on your own.

The staircase has ten steps which will take you down into the vault. I am going to count you down the staircase and with each number that you hear you will start to relax and enjoy the time on your own. Take the first step now.

10: You are starting to go down the staircase – relax
9: Take another step now – relaxing more and more – getting away from being busy
8: Start to enjoy even more the peace and time alone
7: Moving down and away from the busy-ness of the world – slowing down
6: Moving down and away from things or people that have been bothering you
5: Moving down and away from things that have been worrying you
4: Really feeling peaceful now as you step down again
3: Down towards the vault
2: Feeling relaxed and peaceful – slowing down even more
1: Nearly there now
0: Step into the vault.

Walk forward now and explore the vault. The vault stretches out – it goes far and wide underneath the bank – there are corridors going off in all directions. There are doors to different rooms which contain safe deposit boxes. You will see light switches on the wall so you can turn on the lights to make the corridors bright and clear to navigate. There are chairs and tables scattered about for people to use. You can relax here – enjoy the alone time – the peace and the quiet.

Additional script 1: Prioritising

You have a lot going on in your life at the moment. You are so busy – no time to think properly. So much to think about – decisions to be made. It can put you under a lot of pressure – you can sometimes feel that you need to do things quickly. Maybe you have deadlines to meet – maybe other people are badgering you to make a quick decision about something.

Any of this can be very stressful and that is what you do not need – stress. I want you to ask yourself the question; 'Is this really necessary?' – and I want you to regularly repeat the question – 'Is this really necessary?'

You need to slow down – give yourself space – take some time to be alone. You need time to think without any pressure being put on you. You need time to reflect. You then need to prioritise and ask: 'Is this really necessary?' When there is so much going on and you feel pressurised it can feel like things are getting out of control. You need to calmly consider whether you do need to deal with something right at that very moment – maybe it can wait. You need to prioritise what is important for you – not for other people. It is easy to fall into the habit of responding to other people's needs – becoming so busy that you do not consider your own needs – and in fact you neglect yourself.

So now just sit back in a comfy chair in the bank vault. Keep breathing in and out very slowly. Slowing everything down – there is no rush at all. Now start thinking about all the things you are dealing with at the moment – the things that you believe need sorting out right now. I want you to imagine each thing. Now there is a table nearby. When you have thought about everything you need to sort out I want you to place them on the table – in two piles. There is the priority pile and the non-urgent pile. The priority pile is for what does need to be dealt with fairly quickly. The non-urgent pile is for things that can wait.

(Guidance note: the hypnotherapist can continue with the script or if s/he wishes to do more in-depth work some specific questions can be asked as suggested below)

Tell me what you need to deal with.
Which pile will you put that in?
You want to put that in the priority pile – tell me the reason for that.
You want to put that in the non-urgent pile – tell me the reason for that.
What was the reason for thinking this was urgent before now.
You have now prioritised – well done. You have the priority pile and the non-urgent pile. Look at both piles.

(Guidance note: the hypnotherapist should wait for the client to respond to each individual question which follows and discuss)

How big is the priority pile?
Does that surprise you?
How big is the non- urgent pile?
Does that surprise you?
So let's put the non-urgent pile out of the way first – so it is not staring you in the face. There are plenty of safe deposit boxes in the vault – all different sizes. Go and find one which is the right size for the non-urgent pile. Tell me when you have found the right safe deposit box. Now put all the non-urgent things in the safe deposit box and lock them away. How do

you feel now that you realise those things are non-urgent and they have been locked away?

Now have a look at the priority pile. Tell me what is in that pile.
What needs to be dealt with first?
How will you do that?
When will you do that?
What will you deal with next?
How will you do that?
When will you do that?

(Guidance note: continue until the client has gone through the whole pile)

How do you feel now?

(Guidance note: the hypnotherapist should wait for a response and discuss)

You see you do not have to deal with everything immediately. You can slow down – take time to think and reflect – and then decide what really needs to be dealt fairly quickly. Some things can wait and can be put away until you have time to give them your attention. You will think about what is best for you – what you need to give priority to – and what can wait. You will not be pressured by other people. Take time out to be alone – think about you – ask yourself: 'Is this really necessary?' Slow yourself down – you do not need to be busy all the time – slow yourself down. Take your time and ask yourself: 'Is this really necessary?'

Additional script 2: Time corridor to the past

It is time to explore more of the corridors that are down here in the bank vault. The corridors in the vault stretch far and wide underneath the bank and beyond. There are so many corridors – leading to rooms which keep things locked away in safe deposit boxes – really safe. It can be good to unlock things – take them out – and look at them. There are many things locked away in your subconscious mind. When the time is right it is good to unlock those memories. Unlocking some of them could help you deal with *(insert the loss or related issue to be dealt with)*.

Stand up and look around you. You will be aware of one corridor because you entered the vault that way. Take your time and become aware of the other corridors which exist in this area. There are many directions you could go in. You need to find the corridor that will take you back in time – back through your lifetime – this lifetime – and maybe back to a past life. You need to find your own time corridor. Going back in time can help you to remember – help you to understand – release things – memories – thoughts – and very impor-tantly – feelings. Remember along the corridors in the vault there are light switches on the walls to make the corridors bright and clear to navigate. So take a deep breath – look around you – and decide which way you want to go. Start walking now. Find your own time corridor that will take you back in time. Keep walking and walking – along the different corridors – until you find your time corridor. Tell me when you get there and then stop walking. Take your time there is no need to rush. Keep calm and relaxed as you keep walking along.

Good – you have found your time corridor. Make sure the lights are switched on so you can see clearly into your time corridor. You will see that there are lots of doors leading to rooms on this corridor and each room is filled with safe deposit boxes. So get ready to walk down your time corridor – you are going to go back in time. On the count of *3*, you will start to walk down your time corridor – *1, 2*, and *3* – start walking. You are going back in time – back and back – back and back. Look at the doors to the different rooms. Imagine behind the doors all the safe deposit boxes containing your memories. Going back in time – back and back – back and back. When you feel drawn to a particular room let me know and stand outside the door.

Good – you are ready to go into the room. On the count of *3*, you will open the door and walk into the room on your time corridor – *1, 2*, and *3* – go into the room. You see a lot of safe deposit boxes. Which one would you like to open? OK – feel in your pocket and you will find a key. Go and unlock the safe deposit box. Look inside the box and tell me what memory is coming out of the safe deposit box.

(Guidance note: the hypnotherapist then works with the client to relive the memory and release the feelings associated with it. Some prompts and questions follow)

What memory is coming back?
Are you in the memory or looking down on it?
Where are you?
Is anyone else there?
What is happening?
What is being said?
How are you feeling?
What happens next?
Tell me more about that.
Stay with what you are seeing/doing.
Go to the next significant event.
What have you learnt from this?
Do you need to understand anything else?
How are you feeling now?
Are you ready to release that feeling(s)?
Release it now – let it go.
How do you feel now you have released the feeling(s)?
What is different?

(Guidance note: the hypnotherapist can ask the client to open another safe deposit box or return to the room in a future session)

41 Calendars of life

Introduction

This script facilitates regression and is useful when a person who has experienced a loss wants to remember the good and happy times – perhaps from a relationship or situation – rather than focussing on the bad experiences. However, some clients may have regrets and feel they need to look back at what happened. They want to look back and analyse what happened in order to gain some understanding. The script will help them do this. It can also be used to help clients remember things they have forgotten or recall specific events. People who have been bereaved can go through periods of time when they struggle to remember what a person looked liked, what actually happened or when it happened.

The script

It can be good to remember certain times in your life – both good times and perhaps the not so good times. The good times you may remember as happy times and want to relive them. The not so good times may have left you with bad or painful memories, which actually need to be worked on and released. Your subconscious mind is always there to protect you and it may do this by suppressing some memories.

Imagine it is the last day of a year – a time to reflect on the past and also to think about the future. You are sitting at a desk, which has a number of different drawers underneath the top of the desk. This desk stores all the calendars of your life. Just take some deep breaths and let your mind drift back over the years – your lifetime. We are going to ask your subconscious mind to bring forward years – months – days which are significant for you in relation to *(the loss experienced or anything in particular the client wants to address/revisit)*.

Look at the drawers underneath the top of the desk. Each drawer has calendars in it. Which drawer do you want to open? Open that drawer now and look at the calendars in it. Pick the calendars up – feel them – flick

DOI: 10.4324/9781032245706-46

through them. Which calendar do you want to look at? When you have decided place it on the desk in front of you. Look at the calendar.

What year do you see written on the calendar?
What does the calendar look like?
How is it laid out?
What colour is it?
How are the words and numbers written? *(size, font, colour)*
Has it got any pictures?

Take some deep breaths in and out – relaxing – feeling at ease as your mind goes back in time. As you are drifting back the pages on the calendar start to flick backwards and forwards through the months. Watch the pages flick backwards and forwards – they keep flicking backwards and forwards – and then they will stop at some point.

What month is it?
What date or dates are marked in this month?
What happened on this date?
Why is this date important/significant?
What is the reason you need to remember this date?
Tell me more about what happened on this day/at that time?
What do you remember?
What happened then?
What happened next?
How did you feel at the time?
How do you feel now?
What have you learnt from that experience?
Do you need to look for other dates in this calendar?

(Guidance note: if other dates do need to be found then the process is repeated)

Put that calendar to one side now. Do you want to look at any other calendars from that first drawer you opened or do you want to open another drawer?

(Guidance note: if other drawers do need to be opened the script is repeated)

42 Not always what it seems

Introduction

Experiencing a loss can affect how a person sees things and consequently maybe their judgement. A client may become very 'blurred' for a while. They can make assumptions or jump to a conclusion too quickly. These are all very normal reactions and behaviours when dealing with a loss. The main objective of the script is to encourage the client not to respond immediately to what they see (or hear) but rather take time to explore and look deeper into the picture. This is done through imagining and using the 'Death' card in a pack of tarot cards, which is often misinterpreted. The card symbolises an end of something – an era or chapter in one's life – rather than an actual death.

This script is particularly useful for clients who have lost their job unexpectedly and may feel like blaming someone. It is also a very powerful script for when someone has not had good news about some aspect of their health. A person can be in a state a shock when they are first told something and may not hear the rest of the information or advice they are being given.

The script

It is all too easy to jump to a conclusion – maybe think we know best and not listen to anyone else – maybe think in a certain way and not consider other possible interpretations. We think we know what something means, but in fact sometimes a situation is not always what it seems.

I wonder if you have ever seen a pack of tarot cards. Even if you have not, I know you will be able to imagine a pack or even a single tarot card. One of the cards in a pack of tarot cards is known as the death card and people often assume it indicates that a death is going to occur. People can fear getting the death card in a spread of cards. In fact this card does not mean death at all. It actually signifies the end of something but the start of something new. When something does end, there will always be something to follow – a new beginning.

DOI: 10.4324/9781032245706-47

I want you to imagine the death card. The word 'death' is written at the bottom of the card. When people see that word they can jump to the conclusion the card means a death will occur, but remember a situation is not always as it seems. The card signifies the end something – an era – a situation – a relationship – a job – an event – a way of thinking about things – a feeling – a way of responding to things. Above the word 'death' there is a beautiful, strong white horse striding forward. The rider on the horse is proudly carrying a flagpole and a flag is fluttering in the breeze. The horse and rider are striding towards a person in front of them who has their arms stretched out and their hands open – welcoming them to a new beginning.

On the ground there are people and objects that have been left behind. If you look more closely – look around the card – look deep into the card – you will see many other things too – good things. A river – a boat – a cliff – trees – a tower – and behind the tower is a rising sun. It is all too easy just to focus on the word 'death' – you need to look deeper and see the good things that are shown within the card. The river is flowing naturally – the boat can take you on a journey – you can go wherever you want to go. Appreciate the beauty of nature and buildings within the card. Sometimes you need to look hard to find things before you actually see them. Look around the card again and tell me what you see.

It is now time to change things and look to the future. You are going to change the way things are on the tarot card. You have been through a lot lately. You have lost *(insert whatever the client has lost)* – now is the time for a new beginning. The first thing you need to do is strike out the word 'death' on the bottom of the card and insert the words 'new beginning'. Do that now. It is time for you to take the place of the rider on the white horse – climb up onto the horse. The rider passes you the flag. Think about what you would like to see on the flag – what you want it to represent – for the future. What will you have on the flag? *(prompt if necessary: a picture or drawing – sign or symbol – a word – a saying – a mantra)*. Put on the flag whatever needs to be there. Then hold the flag up high.

Before you start going forward on the white horse – look to the ground – see what you are leaving behind. Think about what you have been through – what you have lost – what you are now ready to leave behind. Look at the ground.

What has come to an end already?
What do you want to leave behind?
Who do you want to leave behind?
What needs to come to an end now?

(Guidance note: the hypnotherapist should leave plenty of time for the client to respond to each question)

You can ride forward now into the future – you are ready. Look at the person standing in front of you and the horse – their arms stretched out and their hands open – welcoming you to a new beginning. Look forward – what do want in your future? Whatever you want in the future – place it in the card now. You can make the future just as you want it to be. Tell me what you are placing in the card.

(Guidance note: the hypnotherapist works with the client's aspirations regarding: people; situations; events; feelings)

Now you have made the card just as you want it to be. This is your future – just as you want it to be. New beginnings – you have left the past behind. You need to carry the card with you – place it somewhere safe about your person – so you can bring it out at any time to look at the future and remind yourself about what you want to do – what you want to achieve. Do that now – place it somewhere safe about your person – so you can bring it out at any time to look at the future and remind yourself about what you want to do – what you want to achieve. Just tap where you have placed the card. Remember to always look deeply into things – search for things. Do not make assumptions after taking only a cursory glance. Remember things are not always what they seem.

43 Finding a lost object

Introduction

I am sure everyone can think of a time when they have misplaced something; you know you had it, but have no idea where the thing is now. It can be very frustrating, especially when it is something which is very important. This has happened to me many times but on two occasions quite recently. Firstly, someone needed to see the certificate for my social work qualification. Secondly, I could not find the two spare sets of headphones I keep for delivering webinars. What was so annoying was that both things are always kept in specific places. The social work certificate should have been with all my other certificates, but it was not. I needed to produce the certificate quite urgently, so after hunting high and low I decided I needed to do some self-hypnosis. I have used regression techniques with clients to help them find lost objects, so I thought I needed to do the same for myself. I did go into trance and asked my subconscious to work with me to find the certificate. On coming out of trance I knew exactly where to find the certificate; it was in the strangest of places and I have no idea why I had moved it there. At a later time I also found the headphones, which again had ended up in a very strange place. I did not need to know the reason I had moved these things. I just wanted to find them and I did. So the following script is one that can be used with any client to find an object they have lost.

The script

I know you want to find *(insert object)* and you really want to do this, but for now just relax and do not think about *(object)* right at this moment. It is more important for you to concentrate on relaxing. So just relax – breathe in and out – nice and slowly. Just breathe out any cares, worries or stresses you may have. Things will happen naturally if you let them – do not force anything at all. Breathe in – and then breathe out. Good. Now keep breathing nice and slowly and as you do so, I am going to ask you to imagine certain things.

DOI: 10.4324/9781032245706-48

As you keep breathing nice and slowly, I want you to imagine that you are looking at you when you are standing sideways – so you are in profile. Now look at your head only – a profile view of one side of your head. You can see your hair *(or use 'skin' in place of 'hair' if the client is bald)* which is covering your skull – you can see the side view of your forehead – nose *(put in 'ear' if someone has short hair and it can be seen)* – mouth and chin. Now I want you take away the hair and skin that is covering your head – do that now – so you are looking at your skeleton – your skull. Now see your brain inside your skull. Your clever subconscious mind is in there – there to help you. Have a good look at your brain – walk around – look at it from all angles. Keep looking at the brain. Each side of the brain has four lobes. If you look at the lobes you will see what looks like pathways – bending round. Look deep into the lobes and what looks like pathways.

Your subconscious mind can take you anywhere you want to go – you can have fun just relaxing or going to different places for distraction or for any other purpose. Your subconscious mind knows everything about you. It stores everything you have ever seen, heard or done. So it can help you find *(object)*. It is important to you – you want to find *(object)*. Keep looking at the lobes and pathways in front of you. Now think about *(object)*. You know which lobe you need to enter. Move towards that lobe and enter it now. Choose a pathway to walk along. This pathway is going to take you back in time – it is going to take you back to when you last had *(object)* in your possession. So start walking along the pathway – going back in time to the time when you had *(object)*. Keep walking along the pathway. Keep going back in time – back and back – back and back – until you see you and *(object)*. Back and back you go. Tell me when you see you and *(object)*.

(Guidance note: the hypnotherapist will then work with the client to see what they did with the object and to find where it is now)

Where are you?
What are you doing?
Where is *(object)*?
What happens next?
What happens to *(object)*?
What do you do with *(object)*?
Where is *(object)* now?

44 Layla and the spoon

Introduction

The metaphorical story of Layla is concerning a young girl who is about to be the victim of a forced marriage and can be used for other young people (both female and male) who may be at risk of being force married or are being forced to lead very restricted lives. If a hypnotherapist has little knowledge about forced marriage, I suggest they undertake some specific reading. There are useful links on the Government information website about forced marriage, the Forced Marriage Unit, resources for victims and legislation.[1] It is also useful to read the established multi-agency guidelines.[2] I have experience of working with victims of forced marriage and wrote the story of Layla so I could illustrate the importance of having an anchor. The spoon is the anchor in Layla's story. In order to understand more about why a spoon is a useful tool for people who are at risk of forced marriage, a hypnotherapist should visit the Karma Nirvana website.[3] The story also illustrates the importance of not giving up hope by imagining, planning and rehearsing.

The script

I want to tell you about a girl called Layla, who was 15 years old when she found herself locked up in the loft of her family home. I think you will find the story of Layla very interesting. Layla never gave up – she always had hope. Let me tell you a little bit more about Layla and whilst I am talking about Layla perhaps you would like to imagine her and what happens to her.

Layla was the eldest daughter of Mr and Mrs Ahmed. She lived with her parents, paternal grandmother, her two brothers and two sisters. Layla was a very lively, funny and loyal girl. She respected her parents, but found it hard living by their rules. You see Layla was liked by a lot of people at school because she was friendly and funny; and she was always very open – she said exactly what she thought. Many of her friends came from different backgrounds and cultures. Layla wanted to be what they called

DOI: 10.4324/9781032245706-49

westernised. She liked to dress in trendy clothes, wear make-up, hang out with her friends after school and do things that her parents and grandmother did not approve of at all.

Layla was due to take her GCSEs in May and June. She had her 16th birthday coming up in July which she was really excited about. In March, about a week before the Easter holidays, Mr and Mrs Ahmed told Layla that she was going to be taken to Pakistan. Layla said she did not want to go because she needed to study for her GCSEs. Lots of arguments followed between Layla, her parents and grandmother. Although it was never said, Layla feared that she was going to Pakistan to be married. Layla talked to one of her teachers at school about her fears. Now you might think this very strange but the teacher gave Layla a spoon. She told Layla to keep the spoon hidden in her underclothes. She explained the reason for this. If Layla was taken to an airport, after she had checked-in she would go through security checks in an area where she and her hand luggage would be scanned. The spoon would set off an alarm and she would be able to ask a security person for help.

Layla did keep the spoon hidden – at first in her bedroom. As the arguments at home got more frequent and intense, Layla started to hide the spoon in her underclothes. She knew what had happened to other girls who had been victims of forced marriage. They had been guarded very carefully by family members – they were never left alone – they were walked to and from school. This did not happen to Layla. Her parents decided to lock her in the loft in the house. Layla was locked in there for five days.

Layla was very scared. The loft was a horrible place to be. It was very dark as there was no lighting. She had to sleep on the bare floorboards. She was brought food and drink twice a day. She was not allowed to wash or change her clothes. The days seemed very long. Layla tried to sleep, but she found it hard because she kept thinking about what was going to happen to her. She became very anxious – she felt sick – and sometimes she could not stop shaking.

Layla had the spoon with her in the loft and when she touched it she felt calmer. She would stop feeling anxious and think more positively. She knew she just had to put her hand on the spoon and believe she could get someone to help her. She started imagining going to the airport, checking in and going through the security checks area. She imagined the alarm going off and a security person coming to check her. She rehearsed by imagining what she would say to the man or woman.

Layla started to plan and rehearse in her mind what she was going to do. Every time she did this, she would hold the spoon in her hand. The spoon made her feel calmer – it made her think positively – it gave her hope. The more she imagined – planned – and rehearsed – with the spoon in her hand – the calmer and more positive she became. Imagining, planning and rehearsing helped the time to go quicker.

One morning Mrs Ahmed came into the loft without any food for Layla. She told Layla she could leave the loft, have a shower and put on some clean clothes. After she had done this, Layla was taken with her grandmother to the family car. Mr Ahmed drove Layla and her grandmother to the airport and saw them check-in before he left.

Layla was ready. The spoon was in her underclothes. She sometimes just touched it and she felt hopeful. As Layla and her grandmother queued up to go through customs, Layla imagined what was going to happen – she was ready. The queue was moving very slowly, but with each step Layla felt hopeful. She was getting nearer and nearer to the place where she would put her bag, so it could be scanned by the X-ray machine. The bag started moving as the security person indicated to Layla that she should walk through the machine where she would be scanned. Layla touched the spoon and started to walk forward. Then it happened – the alarm went off.

A security person came towards Layla. She told him she needed help as she thought she was going to be forced into marriage and she said: 'I have a spoon'. The security person knew exactly what this meant and led her to a room for safety. Layla was helped by the airport staff and she did not fly to Pakistan. Layla had never given up. She had hope all through her ordeal. She imagined, planned and rehearsed – and she had her spoon. The spoon helped her to focus – it gave her hope.

Notes

1 Government guidance: https://www.gov.uk/guidance/forced-marriage. Forced marriage Unit, resources and legislation: https://www.gov.uk/stop-forced-marriage.
2 H. M. Government (2014) Multi-agency Practice Guidelines: Handling Cases of Forced Marriage. London: Cabinet Office. https://assets.publishing.service. gov.uk/government/uploads/system/uploads/attachment_data/file/322307/HMG_ MULTI_ AGENCY_PRACTICE_GUIDELINES_v1_180614_FINAL.pdf.
3 https://karmanirvana.org.uk/when-is-a-spoon-not-just-a-spoon/.

45 Wizards

Introduction

We all need a bit magic in our lives and magical things can happen whilst in the trance state. The subconscious mind can do magical things and is a bit of wizard. It is not just children who can enjoy magic, so two versions of the script are presented below. The first script is for a child, who imagines their wizard, gets to know him/her and then is taught how to get rid of unwanted feelings using a wand. The wizard can be used in future sessions to learn more magic tricks in order to deal with issues the child is experiencing. The second script is for an adult and works well for someone who has lost confidence and/or trust in other people.

Script 1: For a child

I wonder what you imagine when you think of a wizard. Do you think of Dumbledore in the Harry Potter books and films or Gandalf in Lord of the Rings or maybe Merlin? Maybe you see an older man with a long white beard, wearing a pointed hat on the top of his head. Wizards are very clever people. They can appear in different disguises. All of them can perform magic – they can do tricks – but they are also very, very wise indeed and can give you good advice when you need it. Everybody has their own wizard and you should always listen to what your wizard has to tell you. Your wizard will always give you very good advice when you need some help with something.

Now I wonder what your very own wizard looks like. I bet you could magic up your wizard now. Imagine that you are standing with a wand in your hand. Start waving the wand about and ask your wizard to appear. Keep waving the wand about and wait for your wizard to appear. *1, 2, and 3* and there's your wizard. Tell me what your wizard looks like.

(Guidance note: on rare occasions a child has imagined an object as the wizard. If this happens the hypnotherapist will need to change the language and use 'it' where s/he or him/her is used in the script)

DOI: 10.4324/9781032245706-50

What is your wizard like?
Is your wizard a man or a woman?
Is your wizard young or old?
What is s/he wearing?

It would be good to get to know your wizard. Introduce yourself to your wizard and ask him/her if they have a name. Have a good chat with your wizard now – get to know your wizard – s/he knows a lot about you already. S/he knows that you have lost *(insert loss)* and you have been feeling *(insert whatever is appropriate for the child)*. The wizard is here to help you. You can always talk to the wizard about how you feel or ask him/her any question. The wizard can also teach you some magic to help you deal with things. You have a wand already. Your wizard has a wand too and s/he can teach you how to do many magical things. It can even make things disappear. You might like to tell your wizard about *(the loss)* and how you have been feeling *(if required insert appropriate feelings for the child e.g. sad, scared, alone, unconfident)*. It would be good to get rid of those feelings wouldn't it? Now watch your wizard – and listen to your wizard – you will learn a lot of useful things. Listen carefully to your wizard –s/he is going to tell you some magic words. Listen carefully now and remember the magic words. Now watch your wizard – look how s/he is waving his/her wand about. Wave your wand in the same way. Good. Now keep watching your wizard and waving your wand. Think about those feelings you want to disappear and at the same time say those magic words and keep waving your wand. Make those feelings disappear. Keep waving the wand until all those feelings have disappeared completely.

Well done. Your wand and the magic words made those feelings disappear. You can feel calm and relaxed now. From this moment onwards you are going to feel so much better. You are going to feel *(insert as appropriate for the child e.g. happy; confident; strong; fearless)*. As each day comes and goes you are going to feel even more *(insert as appropriate for the child e.g. happy; confident; strong; fearless)*. Is there anything else or way you want to feel?

Remember that you can wave your wand to make your wizard appear at any time you need to see him/her or need something magical to happen. You can talk to your wizard about anything. You can ask your wizard questions or for some advice – remember your wizard is very wise. S/he can teach you some more magic too. For now though you have your wand. To make things go away just wave your wand and say the magic words.

Script 2: For an adult

I wonder what you imagine when you think of a wizard. Do you think of Dumbledore in the Harry Potter books and films or Gandalf in Lord of the Rings or maybe Merlin? Maybe you see an older man with a long white beard, wearing a pointed hat on the top of his head. Wizards are very clever people. They can appear in different disguises. All of them can perform magic – they can do tricks – but they are also very, very wise indeed and can give you good advice when you need it. You might think you are bit too old to be thinking about wizards, but everyone has their own wizard and you should always listen to what your wizard has to tell you. Your wizard will always give you very good advice when you need some help with something.

Wizards are everywhere – all around us. Sometimes they are invisible – at other times they pop up when you least expect them. Your wizard will appear when you ask it to or when it thinks you could do with some help or support. Your wizard could appear in many different disguises but remember it is always looking out for you and is there when you need some help. On the count of *3* your wizard is going to appear – I have no idea in what disguise – it will be interesting to find out. *1, 2,* and *3* – and there is your wizard. What is your wizard like?

(Guidance note: the wizard may appear in human form but the hypnotherapist should not be surprised when working with an adult client if the wizard appears in another form e.g. some sort of gadget, machinery. If this happens the script will have to be adapted. The rest of script is written for a human form)

Greet your wizard – thank him/her for appearing – and ask him/her if they have a name. You notice that the wizard is holding a small box in his/her hand. The box is full of messages for you. Remember your wizard knows everything about you – s/he is with you every day – s/he sees and hears what happens to you. Your wizard knows that you have lost *(insert loss)* and that you have been struggling with *(insert difficulties)*. The messages in the box are going to help you – they will give you good advice. The wizard takes the lid off the box and if you look inside you can see lots of bits of paper all folded up. Important messages are written for you on these bits of paper. Take a deep breath and pick a message out of the box. What does it say?

(Guidance note: the hypnotherapist will work with the client to discuss the meaning of the message and how it should be utilised. The hypnotherapist can then choose how to proceed)

Do you want to pick another message out of the box?
Do you want to ask your wizard a question/any questions?

(Guidance note: the hypnotherapist keeps working with the messages for as long as s/he deems necessary for the client)

I think you will agree that the messages you have been given have been very useful. Remember your wizard is always around – often in different disguises – use him/her when you need to do so. For now thank your wizard for helping today – then just relax. You have been given messages to think about and to help you, but for now just relax more and more. Feel more relaxed than you have done for a long while. You have been going through a difficult time, but you are getting through it. Over the next few days and weeks, you will become stronger – you will trust your-self – you will trust your instincts – you will trust other people again. After the next few months you will look back and it will seem magical that you feel so much better and stronger – and *(insert anything else which is appropriate for the client e.g. confident)*.

46 Positivity

Introduction

Experiencing any type of loss can drag a person down into the depths of negativity. A person can sink so low that it feels to them impossible to effect any change. Some clients may never have liked the idea of change and present as resistant. Hypnotherapy is all about enabling and making changes. The following two scripts can be used to help a client think positively – creating both positive thoughts and positive feelings.

Script 1 can work really well in a loss/grief/bereavement group, as it can be read straight through. If working on a one-to-one basis, then the hypnotherapist can ask the client to tell them what they are doing when erasing and multiplying thoughts and feelings. Script 2 embeds the idea that something good can come out of a bad situation. This works well for clients who have a very negative attitude towards everything and the objective is for them to unlearn the habit of seeing everything in a negative way.

Script 1: Signs on the blackboard

Imagine that you are looking at a huge blackboard, which is right in front of you. There is nothing written on the blackboard, but there is some white chalk lying below it and also a chalk eraser. Now you know you can do anything you really want to do, so look at the white chalk and make it rise up towards the blackboard. Look at it hovering ready to write on the blackboard. Now make the chalk draw a big minus sign – then make the chalk write the word 'negative' underneath the minus sign. Good. Now next to the minus sign make the chalk draw a big plus sign and then make the chalk write the word 'positive' underneath it. Good.

Focus your attention on the minus sign. Keep looking at the minus sign. Minus can mean without – a deficit – a loss. Now look at the word underneath the minus sign – 'negative'. Focus on the word 'negative'. Think about the negative thoughts you have been having recently. Let them come into your mind. Let any negative feelings you have been experiencing come into your mind. Stay with those negative thoughts and

DOI: 10.4324/9781032245706-51

feelings. I know it is uncomfortable but stay with those negative thoughts and feelings. As you are thinking about those thoughts and reliving those feelings, make the chalk eraser rise up from where it is lying and make it move towards the minus sign. The eraser is hovering over the minus sign – see the eraser start to rub out the minus sign. Just focus on the negative thoughts you have been having. Watch the eraser rubbing out the minus sign – it is starting to disappear. The negative thoughts start to disappear from your mind. Watch the minus sign disappearing.

(Guidance note: if working with an individual client the hypnotherapist can choose to ask the client to explain what is being erased)

The eraser keeps rubbing out the minus sign – the negative thoughts are still disappearing from your mind – the eraser keeps rubbing at the minus sign until all the negative thoughts have gone completely from your mind. Good.

You can see that part of the minus sign is still left on the board. So now focus on the negative feelings you have been experiencing. The eraser continues to rub at what is left of the minus sign while you are thinking about those feelings. Watch the eraser rubbing out the minus sign – it is disappearing. The feelings you have been experiencing are lessening now – you feel different. The eraser keeps rubbing at the minus sign until all the negative feelings have gone completely from your mind. Good. Look – the minus sign has disappeared completely from the blackboard.

Now focus your attention on the plus sign. Start to think positive thoughts. Think about the future. Let positive thoughts drift into your mind – you know the future can be better than the present. Think about what you want to happen – how you want to feel – what you want to do. As you are thinking these positive thoughts look at the plus sign on the blackboard. Think positive thoughts. As positive thoughts float into your mind, the plus sign starts to get bigger on the blackboard. Let positive thoughts drift into your mind. The plus sign is getting bigger and bigger. Think about what you want to happen – how you want to feel – what you want to do. Look at the plus sign – it is getting bigger and bigger – as more positive thoughts and feelings come into your mind.

(Guidance note: if working with an individual client the hypnotherapist can choose to ask the client to talk about the positive thoughts which are being created)

The plus sign is getting bigger and bigger – you are feeling more and more positive. Really feel those positive feelings. The future is positive – you are positive – you will continue to have positive thoughts – you will continue to have positive feelings. How big can you grow that plus sign? When the plus sign has grown as big as it can on the blackboard – store it in your mind – and anytime you want to think positively or feel positive imagine the plus sign on the blackboard.

Just one more thing to think about. It is good to make more of any positive thing. You can multiply those positive thoughts and positive feelings. Positivity can multiply. So look at the blackboard again and then look for the white chalk. Make the white chalk rise up towards the blackboard. Look at it hovering ready to write on the blackboard. Now make the chalk draw a big cross – a multiplication sign. Then make the chalk write the word 'multiply' underneath the sign. Good. Now think positive thoughts and look at the multiplication sign – feel the positive thoughts multiply. Feel more and more positive thoughts flooding into your mind.

(Guidance note: if working with an individual client the hypnotherapist can choose to ask the client to explain the additional positive thoughts which are being multiplied/created)

I wonder how you are feeling now with all these positive thoughts multiplying in your mind. Concentrate on positive feelings now. Look at the multiplication sign – feel those positive feelings multiply. Enjoy more and more positive feelings inside of you. How positive are you feeling now?

Script 2: Good comes out of bad

When you have experienced a loss and you feel a certain way, it is all too easy to keep thinking negative thoughts. You can dwell on the past – what happened – what was done – what was said – what was not done – what was not said. It can be hard to think positively about the future because you are thinking about the past. Maybe you are thinking: 'Why me?' or 'Why did this have to happen to me?' Whatever happens in your life – good or bad – you will learn something from it. Good comes out of bad and because of that you have got to think differently – you have got to talk differently. You have got to look for the good to come out of a bad experience.

A simple example might be – imagine you are going to take the bus into town. You are running for a bus – you can see it standing at the bus stop. You are running as fast as you can but the driver shuts the door before you get to the bus stop and the bus drives off. You have missed it. Someone else has been running behind you – like you, they needed to catch that bus. The next bus is not due to for another twenty minutes, so you and this person start to walk into town. The good to come out of missing the bus is that you get some unplanned exercise by walking into town, and you have a really good, interesting conversation with someone you have never met before.

A simple example yes – but now let your mind drift back – think of some simple things that have happened to you in your life – in childhood – adolescence – or more recently that maybe were annoying or inconvenient at the time. Just some simple examples – think about what was annoying or inconvenient – then think of any good that came out of the experience. Remember good comes out of bad – you just have to look for it – it may not be obvious at first. Now think back.

(Guidance note: the hypnotherapist should work with the client to identify a number of situations and to talk about them. The following questions can be used to encourage the client to explain in depth what happened and how it affected him/her; before identifying the good that came out of the situation)

What are you remembering?
Tell me what happened.
What were you feeling during that time?
What else do you remember?
What did you learn from that situation/experience?
What good came out of the situation/experience?

So now focus on *(insert the loss experienced)*. I know it has been hard for you and you think of it as a bad thing that has happened. Take a moment now – and try to think of some positives. Think about what you have learnt. Take your time – there is no need to rush. Try to think about the positives. Reflect on what you have experienced and what you have learnt. Think about the positive outcomes.

2 the hypnotherapist should leave plenty of time for the client to think and reflect on their particular loss before focusing on the lessons learnt and encouraging the client to identify the positive outcomes)

Now tell me more about the positives that have come out of this loss.

So now you can see that good can come out of all sorts of situations, can't you? And from now on you will look for the good in all situations, won't you? Your attitude is going to be so positive in the future. You will not be held back by negative thoughts. You know having a positive attitude is much healthier for you. Just as you know something good always comes out of something bad, does it not?

Index

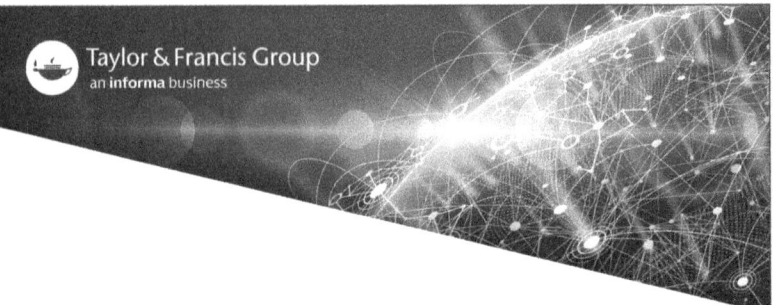
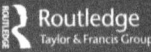
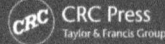